HEALING OUR AUTISTIC CHILDREN

A Medical Plan for Restoring Your Child's Health

HEALING OUR AUTISTIC CHILDREN

A Medical Plan for Restoring Your Child's Health

Julie A. Buckley, MD

with Lynn Vannucci

Foreword by Jenny McCarthy

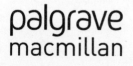

palgrave
macmillan

First published in 2010 by PALGRAVE MACMILLAN® in the United States—a division of St. Martin's Press LLC, 175 Fifth Avenue, New York, NY 10010.

Where this book is distributed in the UK, Europe and the rest of the world, this is by Palgrave Macmillan, a division of Macmillan Publishers Limited, registered in England, company number 785998, of Houndmills, Basingstoke, Hampshire RG21 6XS.

Palgrave Macmillan is the global academic imprint of the above companies and has companies and representatives throughout the world.

Palgrave® and Macmillan® are registered trademarks in the United States, the United Kingdom, Europe and other countries.

ISBN: 978-0-230-61639-4

Library of Congress Cataloging-in-Publication Data
Buckley, Julie A.
    Healing our autistic children : a medical plan for restoring your child's health / by Julie A. Buckley.
        p.   cm.
    Includes bibliographical references and index.
    ISBN 978-0-230-61639-4
    1. Autism in children—Diet therapy.   2. Autism in children—Alternative treatment.   I. Title.
    RJ506.A9B835   2010
    618.92'85882—dc22

                                                    2009020239

A catalogue record of the book is available from the British Library.

Design by Letra Libre

First edition: January 2010
10 9 8 7 6 5 4 3 2 1
Printed in the United States of America.

DEDICATION

For all of the families, including my own, who have had the courage to come into our little "house" in Ponte Vedra.

In search of answers, you have built our community of love, support, and acceptance. Armed with a measure of peace, a breath of hope, and a fount of knowledge, you have gone back out into the wasteland of naysayers, determined to change our world, one child at a time.

The weddings will be fabulous.

CONTENTS

Epilogue
The Longest Marathon

193

ACKNOWLEDGMENTS

Lynn Vannucci, you walked into our lives a veritable autism virgin; you put on, without a second thought, our cloaks of grief, anger, and pain, learned our science, embraced our hope and our determination, and then helped put it on paper, just like that. You amaze me.

Luba Ostashevsky, God bless you for not being insulted when I laughed and was sure that the phone call from the woman who would be my editor was a prank. The entire crew at Palgrave Macmillan has been magnificent. I thought the process was supposed to be arduous and painful?

Jennie Rolfsen, for patiently leading me to the water, and then waiting for me to drink, Dani and I will always be grateful. You saved our lives.

Leslie Weed, for your generosity in teaching me about Lister Hill, Simpsonwood, the politics, and the advocacy, and for showing me how to be a Steel Magnolia through it all, I love your indomitable courage.

Nancy Marin, Bridget Grieco, Eileen Davies, BJ Szwedzinski, Flux Puppy (the newest and youngest therapist), and all of the other members of the extraordinary team who have had a hand in helping to heal my princess, the depth of emotion I feel for you knows no bounds. Thank you for helping me get my little girl back. The marathon continues.

Barb Barton, Brooke Bedwell, Michele Palumbo, Melissa Terbrueggen, Rosie Terbrueggen, and Laurie Thomas—we spend as much or more time with one another than we do with our families, and you make our office a family and a home for our patients. You do the impossible each day with grace and good humor—thanks for making it look so easy.

Jerry Kartzinel, you brought my princess back, returned her future to her. And then you taught me how to do it for others. There are no words.

To my extended family—Bill and Emily Schindler, Tony Pashos, Michelle Harrison, all of the football players who are not just friends, but like adopt-a-sons, all of the folks in my autism world whom I see only every few weeks or months, and the friends and neighbors from our preautism days who have stuck it out with us as we disappeared into the vortex. I am forever grateful for the love and prayers and kinship that are willingly shared, the hearts that are voluntarily opened.

My family—Dean, Matthew, Mom, Uncle Bob—the rest of the world will never know how hard you work and how much you sacrifice. Thank you for your support and patience. Thank you for understanding that I *need* to go 90 miles an hour with my hair on fire. Thank you for understanding how urgently I feel the need to fix this overwhelming problem. Thank you for helping me to try to do it. I love you.

And Dani—my peach. You have worked harder than anyone I'll ever know, are braver than I will ever hope to be. You have gracefully allowed me to share our journey with the world over and over, refusing to be ashamed of what was not your fault and doggedly pursuing normal, whatever that is. You are my hero.

BIOMEDICAL INTERVENTION

HOW TO GET YOUR ODDS ON

To nourish children and raise them against odds is any time, any place, more valuable than to fix bolts in cars or design nuclear weapons.

Marilyn French

Parenthood is the hardest job you will ever love. That's a common sentiment, and lots of people paraphrase it in one way or another all the time. We hear it in the media, and we hear it from politicians, but those of us who are parents know it's not just a platitude. We live the truth of it every day. The difficulties, rewards, challenges, struggles, and outrageous joys of raising happy, well-adjusted, responsible kids are part of our every waking hour—and often part of every sleeping hour too. From the first moment we hold our newborn in our arms, we are consumed with a love that might have previously seemed unaccountable to us. No effort is too exhausting, no sacrifice too grand, no dream too big for our kids.

But when our child is diagnosed with a serious illness, those dreams get deferred. Even derailed. Suddenly, we are dealing with something game-changingly basic—our child's health. The emotions that course through us are primitive: heart-stopping sadness that our worst fears are now confronting us, rage that it is our child who has to suffer, guilt that we are somehow to blame for what has happened. Our brains know that we must be practical, we must get our child treatment, we must *act*—but our hearts are so heavy that focusing on a doctor's often highly scientific explanations and sometimes conflicting information about treatment options can make us feel helpless.

I know this because this is what happened to me when my son, Evan, was diagnosed with autism. My world as I had known it ended, and another very scary world took its place. I had to summon every bit of the courage and toughness it was going to take to learn about his disease, to find the right treatment for Evan and the right doctor to guide us through it, and to become an expert in methylation chemistry, glutathione levels, and chelating agents so that I would always be able to make the right decisions for my son. I had to set aside sorrow and anger and guilt because my son was stuck inside this thing called autism and I had to go there too in order to get him out.

Back in 2005, when Evan was diagnosed, the world of autism was an even more unknown, and therefore scary, place than it is now. Less was known about its causes and treatment—and the appropriate biomedical way to deal with the disease was even less widely accepted in the established medical world. I often compare parents like me, who had to rescue our kids from autism, to the Mom in that old movie *Poltergeist*. We had no idea where our child had gone. The smart, funny, talkative little guy we'd been living with had suddenly disappeared from our home, was being held captive by some inexplicable force, and was being hurt in some way we could not understand; but no matter how terrifying the descent, by God, we were gonna go in there and get him back.

A diagnosis of autism is still a game-changing event for any family. But it is no longer such a mysterious disease. Thanks to the research of brilliant scientists and clinicians, we now know much more about it. We know that it is not a psychological disease at all but a physiological one—and the scientific studies that explain how it affects the body are piling up, offering irrefutable proof that is slowly but ever-more thoroughly being absorbed into standard medical practice. We now have many more physicians and other health care professionals who are trained to offer correct treatment. And we now have a growing base of community knowledge shared on websites and in books as a resource so that we parents are no longer helpless in the face of the inexplicable.

The book you are holding in your hands is one of these incredible resources. It is by Dr. Julie Buckley, the mentoree of Evan's own autistic care specialist, Dr. Jerry Kartzinel. When your child is diagnosed with an autism spectrum disease and you need to understand the science of what is hurting your child, *Healing Our Autistic Children* is the first book you should read. From football games to Jedi Knights, Julie uses vivid analogies that make the often-complicated science clear and comprehensible. In a format that guides you through your first six visits with your autism specialist, she provides you with an easy-to-follow road map through difficult territory you probably never thought you'd have to charter. With a doctor's expertise, a mother's compassion, and a lot of plain old common sense, she describes every tool you'll need to heal your child—and provides the humor and wisdom you'll need to sustain yourself.

Most importantly, Julie has done all of this in a short book that can be a quick read for your harried primary care physician who may not yet be aware of the advances that have been made in the understanding of autism. If your child has been diagnosed with an autism spectrum disease, this is the book to hand to your pediatrician so that he or she can begin to understand the treatment your child needs—and, in the References at the back of the book, he or she will find a listing of the latest scientific research that backs up every step of the biomedical treatment process.

Raising happy, well-adjusted, responsible kids can seem like a long shot to parents of even typical kids. For the longest time, parents of autistic kids were cruelly, and wrongly, told that all bets were off. The information in *Healing Our Autistic Children* helps to even out the odds again for our children. With biomedical intervention, we can rescue them. We can bring them home again whole. And this book is the primer for how we're going to do that.

Jenny McCarthy

INTRODUCTION

GRIDIRON MEDICINE

Once upon a time, there was a little football team. It had the potential to be a good little football team, for it already had many of the basics it would need for success: the appropriate number of players, the right equipment, and a green field on which to play. Moreover, the players themselves possessed varying degrees of raw talent as well as the ambition to win games.

The problem was, at practice every day, the coach concentrated solely on the quarterback. He taught the quarterback all the complicated plays in the playbook, how to hand off seamlessly, and how to throw a long, deep, elegant spiral. The quarterback got pretty good at his job, but the rest of the team ... Well, let's just say there was a lot of chaos out on the field after the ball left the quarterback's hands. The running backs were sluggish from lack of workouts, and the wide receivers couldn't catch, and the coach hadn't taught the plays to anybody else on the team, so there was a great deal of confusion about where the ball was supposed to end up on any given play. Sometimes, because the coach consistently neglected to run blocking drills, a player from the opposing team leaked through the offensive line and sacked the quarterback, before he could even *think* about passing the ball downfield.

Needless to say, this was one terribly frustrated football team. And their fans? Their fans started to call for the coach's head. They wanted to fire that coach and bring in a new coach who could mold the team into an effective, coordinated fighting unit. At the very least, they wanted to bring in someone who could teach the old coach how the game of football was played!

I am a football fan. In addition to being a board-certified pediatrician who specializes in the treatment of autism spectrum diseases (ASDs), I am the personal physician to several NFL players. I never miss one of my team's games. I'm cheering in the stands for every home contest, and I'm parked, along with the members of my whole extended family, in front of the television set on the days our team is away, shouting long-distance encouragement to my guys. For me, football is a way of life—and it is also a terrifically apt metaphor for the successful treatment of ASDs.

Think, for a moment, of the body as a football team. The brain is the quarterback, responsible for telling the rest of the body what to do and how to behave. The digestive tract—the stomach, the intestine, the bowel—is the offensive line, charged with blocking and breaking down food into its component nutrients so that the body can use them most efficiently and eliminate what is no longer useful. The blood and its cells are the running backs, delivering useful nutrients and enzymes throughout the body so that they can be used to construct healthy bones and muscles and be chemically transformed into necessary hormones and antioxidants. Our receptor cells are like biological wide receivers, catching the neurotransmitters thrown from the brain, together with the nourishment tossed to them from the bloodstream. On the defensive side, the immune system is designed to tackle invading forces such as harmful bacteria and viruses and send them packing before they reach the end zone and score. When the team is an effective fighting unit, with each player doing their job to the best of their ability, the body is able to turn in peak performances. If any of these players is injured, however, and unable to coordinate their efforts with the other members of the team, the body ceases to function well. A child with autism is like that team—his body becomes frustrated, falling into physical as well as mental decline because it can't do what it is supposed to do. The fans become frustrated in turn, often depressed or angry, because they intuitively know how great their team could be if only some coach could be found to help the players learn how to correctly execute the game. The fans, in the case of my pediatric practice, are the parents who watch beloved children stumble and struggle as they try to play the game of life under the cloak of autism.

For too long, ASDs have been thought of as mental disorders. The only accepted treatment offered by the medical community for autism has been therapy—occupational, physical, speech, and, in particular, applied behavior analysis (ABA). ABA is a treatment that focuses on retraining the brain so that the autistic patient's behavior becomes more controllable and socially acceptable.

But, as I've just illustrated, no single body can play a winning game if all the team members aren't playing *together*.

While autistic kids may *seem* to suffer from mental distress, their disease is almost invariably accompanied by real physical illness—immune disorders, bowel dysfunctions, and the nutrient deficiencies that cause their bodies to fail in these and other ways. These children are shunted to psychiatrists and therapists because we have so long pegged autism as a mental disorder. Their accompanying medical illnesses remain largely untreated because autistic kids frequently lack the verbal skills necessary to complain that they are in pain. Many of the kids, consequently, turn to self-injury—head banging, scratching, and worse—to assuage their suffering. It is unconscionable to me, as a physician who has sworn to do no harm, that the medical establishment rarely treats the underlying biomedical problems. It is a matter of simple human compassion to provide the appropriate medical care that can bring these children relief from their pain.

Medical schools and hospitals teach that there is no treatment for autism. For them, recovery flies in the face of the current medical model. And yet, in case after case after case, the recovery of autistic children is exactly what happens when their gastrointestinal problems are addressed, for example, and their physical systems are normalized.

Frankly, it eludes me how a doctor, a person who was once trained in the sublimely intricate and intertwined processes of the human body, could fail to comprehend the connection between fixing a child's compromised immune system or irritable bowel and all of a child's systems beginning to function more harmoniously. Let's put this connection in terms all of us can vividly, and immediately, understand.

Have you ever gotten home after a hard day at work and poured yourself a drink? Your glass of merlot or your frosty mug of beer tastes good and feels relaxing. This is because the alcohol in the liquid you're ingesting is interacting with and impacting your body's biological and chemical cycles.

Depending on how much you have to drink, and on your body's tolerance for alcohol, you might begin to talk more freely after a libation or two, slur your words, or even, dare we say, stumble when you attempt to walk. The connection in this instance between the gut (what you are imbibing) and the brain (the impaired judgment that results from your tipple) is so wholly accepted that it is, of course, illegal to drive a car after a certain amount of consumption.

How is it possible that anyone who has ever walked into a bar could deny the intimate relationship between the gut and the brain?

For parents of autistic children, it is most often a matter of common sense that when an autistic system is no longer besieged—no longer required to direct so much of its limited resources to propping up a weakened physical body—the whole child can begin to heal. The fog the child has seemed to live under begins to lift. He stops throwing tantrums, and there is no more need for a helmet to keep him from injuring himself. She sleeps through the night. His need to stim—that is, to engage in repetitive self-stimulating behaviors like hand flapping or hair twirling—lessens. She regains the social, motor, and verbal skills that had been lost. His teachers start to comment on how well he's doing in the classroom. She once again takes an interest in typical childhood play. He once again seeks you out for a hug and says, "I love you." To return to the football analogy, when the coach—the doctor, in this case—stops putting all of his attention on the quarterback—the brain—and starts to focus on bringing the other players in the game up to speed, the team suddenly starts to win games again. With continued intervention, the team earns a playoff berth. The team trains hard, and the fans start to buzz that the Super Bowl is no longer a pipe dream but is actually within reach!

The process of making the Super Bowl a possibility—a *probability*—is called *biomedical intervention*.

For the purposes of this book, I am going to sidestep the controversies that surround the *causes* of autism. Early treatment is essential in the potential recovery of an autistic child, and, like you, I have no desire to be distracted by a shouting match with the medical establishment, which sees biomedical intervention in the treatment of autism as controversial enough. Let me take a moment of your time, however, to touch upon how medical debates can work themselves out, and once far-out ideas can become conventional wisdom.

In our current century, we are still seeing tests and trials and testimonies surrounding the link between tobacco use and cancer. When did the medical establishment know that tobacco was harmful to a person's health? How far did tobacco marketers go to undermine the general dissemination of this knowledge? What interests stood in the way of acceptance of the now-indisputable fact that smoking or chewing tobacco can kill you?

While it may seem as if we've come rather recently to this consensus—because we've only relatively recently come to act upon our knowledge with smoking bans and age-based sales restrictions—it was way back in 1959 that a surgeon general report implicated smoking as a cause of disease. But even that 1959 report wasn't the first time the link was recognized. As long ago as 1761, a London physician, John Hill, published a medical paper, "Cautions against the Immoderate Use of Snuff," claiming that "snuff is able to produce ... swelling and excrescences." By excrescences, he was referring to cancers of the nose. In the United States in the mid-nineteenth century, when tobacco was a tremendous growth industry, New Englander Samuel Green, in the *New England Almanack and Farmer's Friend,* connected the dots between death from lung disease and tobacco smoking. "How is it possible to be otherwise?" he asked. "Tobacco is a poison. A man will die of an infusion of tobacco as of a shot through the head." And in 1928, a paper published in the New England Journal of Medicine by Drs. Herbert L. Lombard and Carl B. Doering, "Cancer Studies ... Habits, Characteristics and Environment of Individuals With and Without Cancer," carried the warning that "the use of tobacco has long been considered a fact in the incidence of cancer."

Still, as late as 1957, a Dr. Harry S. N. Greene was able to write in a popular book, *Science Looks at Smoking,* without fear of becoming a laughingstock: "The evidence (both statistical and experimental) does not appear sufficiently significant to me to warrant forsaking the pleasure of smoking."

In our current century, the medical establishment repeatedly points to the still-meager number of studies that have been funded to learn how biomedical intervention impacts autism. In this way they bolster their argument that the evidence (both statistical and experimental) does not appear sufficiently significant to warrant the use of the techniques of biomedical intervention in the treatment of autism.

How many people died of lung disease because doctors like Harry S. N. Greene refused to see what was right before their very eyes? People were smoking, and these same people were getting sick and dying. This thing they saw right before them looked like a duck. It quacked like a duck. It waddled like a duck. But they still refused to call it a duck.

My point, at the end of all this talk of tobacco, is that more and more kids are today being diagnosed as autistic. But these sick kids are getting better through the use of biomedical intervention. I, and many doctors like me who treat these kids biomedically, see the healing happening every day, with our own eyes. And it looks like a duck to us. It quacks like a duck. It waddles like a duck. So, damn it, we're going to call it a duck, because our kids don't have half a century or more to wait until the statistical and experimental evidence becomes indisputable. Our kids can't wait until conventional fact and the state of medical science catch up to them. Our kids don't have the luxury of hanging on until they get to the right side of history on this one.

So, in this book, I am going to avoid the *why* of autism as much as it is possible to do that and still provide you with a medically cohesive explanation for *how* biomedical intervention works. I am simply going to tell you what I know as a physician—and as the mother of an autistic child and an oppositional defiant child who have both had tremendous recovery through biomedical intervention. I am simply going to tell you the truth, so that you can help your own child to recover *now*.

For purposes of clarity, I've structured this book as a series of six visits to your autism doctor, detailing in each subsequent visit the ways in which you can expect biomedical intervention to progress. Keep in mind that autism is a spectrum disease—we love to point out that "if you've met one child with autism, well, you've met one child with autism." Each child is afflicted differently; their symptoms are tremendously variable in quality and quantity. It should come as no surprise, then, that their progress with treatment will vary tremendously, and that what works well for one child may not work at all for another. Inconvenient, but true. There are, however, some common facts all parents can take to the bank. These are the five brave, basic truths about autism:

1. Autism is a medical illness. It only *looks* like a psychiatric disorder.

2. Autism, as well as those disorders such as attention deficit disorder (ADD), oppositional defiant disorder (ODD), pervasive developmental disorder–not otherwise specified (PDD-NOS), Asperger's syndrome, and a range of learning disabilities that fall on the autism spectrum, is treatable. The foundation for treatment rests in proper diet and nutritional supplementation.

3. Autism is a series of vicious biological and chemical cycles gone awry within the child's body. These cycles interact, impacting immune function, gut function, and methylation chemistry, among other biological systems. (I am going to tell you enough about the chemistry involved so that when you hand this book to your physician and tell him, "Read this. This is the way we're going to help my kid," you can point him toward the appropriate scientific research that backs it up.)

4. Breaking the vicious cycles at the cellular level and normalizing the function of your child's systems is what biomedical intervention is all about.

5. There are safe and effective starting points for each step of the biomedical intervention process (and by the time you are through reading this book, you will know what they are, so you can be a highly effective partner to your child as she recovers).

You'll note that I cast us parents as partners—or "fans"—in our child's recovery. I do this deliberately, for while the process of biomedical intervention may seem initially as if it's a lot of work for the caregiver of an autistic child, it is always the case that the child is the one doing the bulk of the work. We parents may seem like the heroes, but it's our kids who suffer the physical pain and who struggle intellectually and emotionally to emerge from the fog of autism, regain their skills, and lead normal lives. Each day without stimming, every vocabulary word learned, every day with a normal poop—these are rewards that make the process of biomedical intervention joyfully worthwhile for a parent, but they are really our kids' victories.

Remember, as you travel the road to recovery, to celebrate them.

My family? We celebrate by going to another football game.

WHAT IS AUTISM?

THE SEARCH FOR ACCEPTABLE SOLUTIONS

ANGIE I

The first time I met Angie, in 2004, she was ten years old. She was a bloated little girl, carrying far too much weight on her slender bones, suffering from both a thyroid condition and chronic constipation. Her big brown eyes were rimmed with dark circles of fatigue, and they were opened painfully wide, staring through me as I tried to talk with her. She didn't flit around my office, throw herself on the examination table, and then stomp on the scale on the opposite side of the room, uncontrollably in motion like so many of the kids who come to see me for the first time; Angie knew what was expected of her in a social situation because her mother, Carole, had worked for years to teach her. Angie exercised some self-control, but she had no ability to express herself beyond her most basic needs, no depth of language or real social skills. Because of this dearth of language, her doctors and teachers assumed she was mentally impaired. Angie was a student at a special needs program in a Catholic school; in my office she stimmed by systematically shredding, thread by thread, her plaid school uniform.

But of all the symptoms of autism Angie displayed that day in my office, the one that broke my heart—and that continues to consistently break my heart—was the flat, expressionless look on her face. This was a child for whom the world was such a closed and scary place she could experience very few of its pleasures. She could, in fact, react to little at all in the world around her, except with fear. There was no joy in her eyes.

The psychiatrist Leo Kanner was one of the first physicians to recognize and describe a then-emerging condition: autism. In 1943, Kanner wrote a seminal paper, "Autistic Disturbances of Affective Contact," that, together with the work of Hans Asperger, formed the basis for the modern-day study of autism. In that paper Kanner wrote that one of the five-year-old boys he studied at the time, Donald, seemed "happiest when he was alone . . . diving into a shell and living within himself . . . oblivious to everything around him." Though the clinical definition of autism continued to evolve and grow over the ensuing decades, Kanner's early observation goes right to the heart of the disease. The inability of an autistic child to willingly engage emotionally—empathetically—with the world around him remains the classic symptom of true autism. These children are so absorbed within the urgent necessity of their own rituals that they are oblivious to the joy of and delight in discovery that most children take for granted. This absence of wonder is a large part of what has long mired autism in a psychiatric diagnosis—it *looks* as if the child is withdrawn, even absent. But it is also what makes it imperative to treat these children with the wide range of nonpsychiatric techniques now available to help them to heal. It is only a *perceived* lack of wonder we see on these small, blank faces.

I remember looking at Angie that first day, trying so hard to connect with her, because what I had come to know was that there was every possibility a lively mind was trapped within this child's very sick body, hungering for the words she could use to express herself, aching for relief.

However sorry the shape Angie was in that first day I met her, her mother assured me I was not seeing the worst of it. A few months before, Angie's symptoms had been even more profound. This had been a child for whom visual and auditory sensations were so overwhelmingly painful she'd banged her head repeatedly—brutally—against any hard surface she could find in a pathetic, fearsome attempt to dissipate them. She'd had to wear a helmet to keep from injuring herself. It was alarming behavior, and, as Angie got older, it became even more frightening.

As Angie grew bigger and stronger, her mother was less able to control her and, therefore, less able to protect her. She was more fearful of the harm Angie might inflict upon herself as she became an adult. Angie's doctors and teachers were already hard at work preparing Angie's mother to accept the fact that her daughter would soon have to be institutionalized.

In desperation—the sort of expansive fearlessness that can be provoked only by love—Carole had gone looking for answers she wasn't getting in the doctors' offices. She had done what, a scant year before, I myself might have cautioned her against doing: she got on the Internet and Googled for a ray of hope.

What she found on the Net was information about how a gluten-free, casein-free (GFCF) diet could help autistic kids recover. Along the way, she also found that various official agencies, such as the Centers for Disease Control (CDC) and the American Academy of Pediatrics (AAP), were adamant that there was no scientific evidence that such a diet would do any good. Elsewhere, at a site she'd believed belonged to an autistic advocacy organization, the Association for Science in Autism Treatment (ASAT), she found outright condescension for the desperate parent who invested hope in such a diet, a treatment ASAT dismissed as "pseudoscience." But Angie's mother felt her back was up against the wall. Any parent would recoil at the thought of losing her or his child to an institution, and with that unacceptable step as the looming alternative, Carole started her daughter on a nutritional regimen that removed all gluten (essentially wheat, oat, rye, and barley) and casein (essentially anything that comes from an udder) from her diet.

The change in Angie was "miraculous," according to the family. The child was still profoundly autistic, but the worst of her self-injurious behavior had ceased. This was proof enough for Carole that there was something to this diet, and she began to seek out a doctor who could explain to her what it was—who would be able to take the healing to another level and recommend other therapies that could offer the child even greater relief. Angie's family's circumstances were modest, and insurance was certainly not going to willingly foot much of the bill for treatments that were not wholly embraced by the existing medical establishment, but no matter. Sacrifices would be made if there was a chance of releasing her child from the grip of autism.

The unconditional willingness to sacrifice for a child's sake is something I witness every day in the parents who come to see me. It is often in assuring me that there is nothing they will not do to have their child returned to them whole that the parents will begin to cry, and at times like these, I often have to check my own tears. This is the best and the worst of my job. I know what the parents of my patients are feeling. I have lived it, and I relive it with every one of them.

DANI I

In August 2003, within days of receiving her booster vaccinations, my fabulous four-year-old daughter, Dani, disappeared before my very eyes. The child left behind in her body was a stranger to us. Our cheerful little princess came to consciousness each morning moaning and crying. Our chatterbox stopped speaking. Our songbird no longer lifted her voice to serenade us with her favorite ditties—"Twinkle, Twinkle Little Star" and "Tigger's Song." Our daddy's girl no longer wanted to pray at bedtime with her father. She had meltdowns, a new phenomenon in our home, for no discernable reason. If she didn't want to do whatever it was that we wanted her to do, she flopped on the floor like a wet noodle. She cared nothing for being with us—I could leave the house, and she did not notice; I could return, and she did not care. This abrupt verbal and social regression was accompanied by what was, in my mind, at the time, the unaccountable: a brutal bowel disorder that distended and swelled her belly and made her look pregnant. And that frequently resulted in orange diarrhea flung on the walls of our home.

Had I not known this child prior to her regression—had I, for instance, been a new teacher in her classroom—I might have decided that Dani was only a sullen, disagreeable little girl. Had I not known the extensive vocabulary and other accelerated skills Dani had possessed just before she got sick, I might have chalked up her inabilities to her being a little "slow." Had I myself not been recuperating from back surgery during just this same period of time—in other words, had I not been a stay-at-home mom who witnessed firsthand every frightening new loss that accompanied my child's regression—I might have blamed Dani's new willfulness on a lack of discipline in the home. Even as I saw new problems surface each day, I buried myself deeply in that delightfully protective defense mechanism: denial. I refused to see what was clearly present in our house. In the end, I made my husband say it first: autism.

The parent in me couldn't admit it, but as a doctor, I have to make diagnoses such as these daily. A doctor's job can, in many ways, be likened to that of a medical detective. For our clues, we rely on observable signs and symptoms—on behaviors, as well as rashes and swelling, fevers, and the like; on verbal accounts of the illness from the patient and the family histories we ask patients to provide in such detail; on laboratory results we order from blood draws, urine samples, and biopsies; and on the results of tests such as MRIs and CT scans. Modern medical science has provided us with a large toolbox to turn to in gathering our clues. When we have our clues in hand, however, we routinely pick up our textbooks for a little old-fashioned reading and research to help us in confirming a diagnosis and instituting effective treatment.

When Dani got sick, and I at last accepted that her sickness was indeed autism, I turned to my textbooks. You see, back then, I was not a specialist in autism; I was a typical pediatrician taking care of mostly well children—treating earaches and sore throats, and performing annual physical exams. In my textbooks I found nothing that would help me learn about autism save one short paragraph discussing autistic features in some chromosomal disorders. I next hunted through medical literature, but I found nothing that told me how to fix my daughter's problem. What I found instead was that the medical community, of which I was myself an active member, officially considered autism a dead-end diagnosis.

That's when I did what any parent would do: I became furious at a world that would write off my formerly bright, cheerful child as hopeless. I did the thing that as a pediatrician I had routinely cautioned my patients' parents not to do: I Googled my child's illness in the hope of finding helpful information that the outlets of established medical science could not provide or were not providing to me.

What I found, when I Googled autism, were the same sorts of things that Angie's mother, Carole, found when she was looking for answers. But for me, these discoveries generated tremendous internal turmoil between my brain and my heart and between my medical career and my motherhood. What I found at my traditional mainstream medical sites was exactly nothing to help my princess. What I found at places such as the Autism Research Institute was in direct conflict with my medical training: autism was not a psychiatric disorder at all, but a physical illness, and in treating it as such there was hope for recovery. There was a coalescing group of researchers and clinicians calling their approach "Defeat Autism Now!" and they were doing exactly that with a scientific approach to the illness as they understood it. The foundation of Dani's treatment would lie in changing her diet, and supplementating her diet with missing ingredients to repair her weakened physical body.

Now, this made sense to me because of what I was seeing at home. Dani's chronic diarrhea was clear evidence that something was wrong with her digestive system. The fact that she was constantly sick with complicated colds and earaches and other "typical" childhood illnesses indicated that her immune system was distressed. Perhaps—just perhaps—in attending to the very real medical problems that had manifested at the same time as her verbal and social regression, her "mental" problems could also be impacted positively. Remember the gut-brain connection we've already talked about as it relates to the consumption of alcohol? I wondered: Was it possible that by cleaning up Dani's system—by removing those elements from her diet that researchers were finding were toxic to autistic kids (gluten and casein) and bolstering those elements (vitamins and minerals) that were lacking—we could actually help her brain to clear too?

So, early in 2003, we set off, as a family, on this journey into the unknown, and we did it with gusto. We dropped everything else, and Dani did too. We emptied the pantry of the products that would offend Dani's system and learned a completely new way to cook. We gave her the most god-awful tasting mixtures of vitamins and minerals and supplements twice daily. We drew blood, gave infusions, and eliminated the yeast in her diet (the impact of which on the digestive system I'll explain in detail later), detoxifying her under the guidance of Jerry Kartzinel, a brilliant clinician who already had broad experience working with the biomedical recovery of autistic kids—and who mentored me as I learned the science.

The process of detoxification was a roller coaster. Our family was anguished when Dani was kicked out of her first school because the symptoms of withdrawal from gluten and casein, no matter that they were transient, were so severe. We watched with pride at her determination to get well; she worked her fanny off day after day, attending seven hours of different therapies over the course of every five workdays—and this after putting in a full day at school. Though her social skills still needed work, and though her body still needed a great deal of support, in a relatively short 18 months she had regained 47 IQ points, was labeled as gifted, and was mainstreamed at her new school.

We were blessed.

And I knew I had found my calling: to help other families experience the same blessing of recovery.

ONE IN SIX

I suspect that I would never have put significant effort into learning how to treat a child with autism if I hadn't been compelled by Dani's illness. That's because biomedical intervention is not a magic bullet. There is no single pill to prescribe, no one shot to give. You've just read a little bit about Dani's story, and it sounded short and sweet, with a neat, happy ending. But read it again. Dani's initial recovery extended over a hard-fought 18 months, and even today, five years later, her body still requires nutritional support, and she still needs help navigating the complex social world of typical preadolescent girls. Learning how to support Dani and manage her illness was required of me as a mother; it was a no-brainer. However, as a physician, learning to manage a complex disease such as autism, long after my training years were behind me, would have been professionally unappealing, and even inefficient. As a primary care pediatrician, it would have made more sense simply to refer a child who presented with autism in my practice to a specialist.

Wouldn't it?

When I started to look for information that would help me to treat Dani, I was astonished that there really was an extensive amount of published literature on what was wrong with her and how to fix it. There is a tremendously talented group of brilliant researchers and experienced clinicians working on solutions.

When Bernie Rimland, PhD, gathered Jon Pangborn, PhD, and Sid Baker, MD, together asking for help to solve the autism problem as he understood it, they set out in search of a few "really smart people" to think about it. Today, those people are much like a family, spanning the globe, located in both private practices and universities. From Martha Herbert, MD, PhD, at Harvard and Dick Deth, PhD, at Northeastern, to Jill James, PhD, at the University of Arkansas, and a host of others around the world, researchers are sharing their findings with incredible clinicians like Anju Usman, MD, Ken Bock, MD, Nancy O'Hara, MD, Stu Freedenfeld, MD, Liz Mumper, MD, and Mary Megson, MD, to name just a few. These clinicians, collaborating with "bench" researchers—those scientists who spend the predominance of their time not with patients but in the lab—are implementing findings in real time, *now*, in children with autism.

At first, I was surprised and delighted to find such a wealth of resources, but the thrill of discovery quickly turned to disgust and anger: Why *hadn't* any of this material been covered in medical school? How was it possible that as a young pediatrician, I hadn't been exposed to at least some of this material in the classroom? That's when the horrible truth hit me: I hadn't been taught this material because medical schools weren't teaching it. If this knowledge about biomedical intervention wasn't available in school, where did I think these autism specialists were going to come from? Soon enough, however, I had to put all emotion aside and rehone my skills at acquiring medical knowledge. Gaining a working understanding of how to treat autism was going to be daunting. I knew I wouldn't have the energy to do it if I stayed inside my anger.

I essentially went back to residency all over again. I did it at night in bed, devouring articles and relearning detested biochemistry. I worked up essays, drew diagrams, and found analogies, wending my way through this complex and evolving medicine. Through all this my husband was infinitely patient. The light by my side of the bed burned late into the night; I often talked medicine in my sleep; and when my husband woke up in the mornings, he faced a wife whose eyes were slits and whose usual cheery "Good morning!" was reduced to a groan for a cup of coffee.

The hard work paid off; I am now considered an expert in the world of autism, working with children and mentoring clinicians from all corners of the globe.

But remember what I said about being motivated to become an expert because my daughter needed me to do that? The need is no less urgent for parents who are not physicians, but who still have to care for an autistic child.

There is today a tremendous disconnect between obtainable knowledge and implemented treatment for autism. There is an ever-widening gap between what parents know and what physicians know. The parents have made themselves experts in complex bio-chemistry, immunology, and gastroenterology. They know what is happening on the cutting edge of autism treatment because their kids need them to know. This kind of parent overtakes their pediatrician's expertise very quickly.

This is infuriating to me. There is nearly a three-year waiting list for a child with autism to come see me. Twelve- to fourteen-hour workdays moving like I'm on roller blades and my hair is on fire are routine. There are quite a few experienced specialists in my field now, and they all have work schedules and waiting lists like mine.

Why?

The statistics for young children who have been diagnosed with autism are carefully charted by the Centers for Disease Control (CDC). In 2008, those statistics were 1 in 150 in the United States, and 1 in 100 in Britain; four out of five patients are boys. In August, 2009, the CDC revised those statistics—upward: the cases of autism in the United States are now 1 in 100 too. That means that out of every 10,000 children born in the United States, 100 of them will become victims. But even this sobering statistical increase is not the worst of it. "1 in 100" refers only to cases of "true autism"—to children as profoundly affected as Angie and Dani. When we include the number of children who are diagnosed with other disorders that fall on the autism spectrum—ADD, ODD, PDD-NOS, Asperger's, and other learning disabilities—the number of children diagnosed with ASD is one in six.

One in six.

Take a drive down any suburban street in the nation—perhaps *your* suburban street—at around three o'clock on any weekday afternoon. Watch the yellow buses pull into their stops and see the kids pile off after their school day is over. Count them. Maybe there are 30 kids living in your neighborhood, if your neighborhood is anything like mine. Statistically, five of them are likely to have an autism-related disorder.

Five.

He might be the skittish boy who can't pay attention in the classroom and is now failing third grade. Or she might be the huffy girl who answers back so aggressively when her teacher tries to correct her that she's been suspended twice already this year, and it's only October. He might be sweet and endearing—you know this even though you're his parent and you are patently prejudiced—but the other kids in his fifth-grade class mock him because he's got a signature set of tics he can't control, and it breaks your heart.

You get the idea.

When I was in residency, children who were diagnosed with autism were rare, an oddity; this might go a short way toward explaining why we weren't taught about autism in medical school *then. Now,* one in six kids is afflicted. We have an epidemic of children with a regressive, multisystem illness in which immune systems, guts, brains, and, in fact, whole bodies are quite ill. These children live in some greater or lesser degree of pain that they've had, most of them, since the time when their memory begins. And yet the name given to their illness is classified only in the psychiatric division of medicine. One in six children in one of the wealthiest and most powerful nations in the world do not receive medically appropriate care. If we continue to pretend that ASDs are psychiatric disorders, one in six children will remain medically homeless from a treatment standpoint.

And *that* is what is infuriating.

The supply end of the equation (the lack of experienced clinicians who can treat these kids) coupled with the demand (the astonishing number of children who are suffering) is driving the treatment crisis.

My primary care pediatric peers have said in a recent survey that they feel unqualified and uneducated as to what to do. My Defeat Autism Now! peers are falling over themselves with willingness to teach these doctors what they know. The reason the gap is not being bridged is because of the endless posturing of groups who insist that this epidemic is genetic (a medical impossibility, as you will see as you read on), or a matter of better diagnosis (which would assume that the rates of the other diseases we used to call autism should be going down, and they're not) or the broadened criteria by which we now diagnose the disease ("So if we narrow it," as I've heard Jerry Kartzinel say so many times, "then all these kids will go away?"). For crying out loud! At what point do we finally say "Enough!"? I feel a little like Dorothy must have when Toto pulled back the curtain in *The Wizard of Oz*. You can tell me to "pay no attention to the man behind the curtain" all you want; I still see him. As a parent, I'm looking for answers to what happened to my child, and no matter who tells me that I'm looking in the wrong place, I'm going to leave no stone unturned. As a physician, I think all of us primary care people are going to have to get busy and start trying to figure out how to help the children. If we keep waiting for the great and powerful wizard to tell us how to do it, we may never get our families back to Kansas.

The saving grace in this cause and treatment debacle is going to be parents. The understanding of autism as a treatable, recoverable physical illness is parent led and parent driven. Parents are so far ahead of the medical field in understanding the scope of their children's illnesses that catching up is an embarrassing effort for us physicians.

But eating a slice or two of humble pie should be nothing to us compared to the lives we can save.

As Angie's mother and I began to work together that first year, 2004, she came to each visit armed with a whole list of subjects ready to discuss: killing yeast, glutathione infusions, augmenting and balancing vitamin supplements, hyperbaric therapy, chelation . . . She had found a whole menu of options on the Internet that might hasten her daughter's treatment. She always did her homework. Thankfully, I was also doing mine, and together we guided Angie's recovery. Over the years, Carole and I have taught each other. This reciprocal education is a phenomenon I've celebrated with nearly every one of my patients and their families as, together, we continue to learn about a relatively new and evolving field of medicine and begin the work of healing our kids.

OBSERVE, EXAMINE, ASK, AND EXPLAIN

When a child comes into my office for the first time, he and his parents stay for a minimum of two hours while I observe, examine, ask, and explain.

My office sits immediately opposite my waiting room, and I rarely close the office door. The door is closed, in fact, only when I'm on a telephone consultation with a parent. This is because it is usually painful for any child to sit still for two whole hours, more so for autistic kids; most of them prefer to be in my waiting room, surrounded by stuffed animals, picture books, and the wooden train village that sits in the middle of the room. You might think I leave my office door open so that parents can keep an eye on their child while we're conferring, but there is a more profound method to my madness. With the door open, I too can keep an eye on the child while I talk with her parents. I can see how she behaves over the course of two hours. Does she stim, and how often? Does he line up all the train cars in neat lines? How does she interact with other children who are waiting with their own parents for their infusion treatments or hyperbaric appointments? How does he respond to the members of my staff who pass through the room and greet him? When I begin the physical examination, does she allow me to weigh her and check her height, or does she object? *How* does she object?

I carry out this observation and a basic medical examination while I'm typing notes into the child's file on my computer, asking her parents in-depth questions about their family medical history as well as the history of their child's specific illness. When did they first notice their child's symptoms? How many words did their child have in her vocabulary before the regression began? Or did language never progress at all? And then we move on to my "favorite" topic: we have an extensive discussion about bowel movements. Sometimes getting the first accurate description of poop is horrifyingly embarrassing to families. Sometimes they're shocked to have someone who actually wants all the details. How many times a day does the child go? What is the color of the poop? The consistency? Does it go in the potty or a pull-up? Is it shaped like goat pellets, or is it so voluminous that mom can wield a plunger like a weapon? What does it smell like—the unpleasant odor of normal waste, or is it that death-defying smell that makes the neighbors consider calling HazMat when you open the window to air out the house?

The parents also ask questions during this time, and I answer them, of course, but I've got other items on my agenda, and the appointment continues for as long as it takes for us to cover all of them. I'm gathering my clues, you see, and I love the detecting part of medicine. Among the first things I'll need to do is to have one of my nurses draw the child's blood while the child is here in the office, and I'll need the parents to collect both urine and stool samples to send to the laboratory for analysis.

But, every bit as important as collecting my clues, the child, the parents, my staff, and I need this time to form the beginnings of our therapeutic bond. Together, we are going to create a team to improve this child's health, decrease his pain, and give him back the joy of childhood. In order to do that effectively, it's imperative that we spend some time to get to know one another.

And it's important that we're all on the same page about the science of the child's disease. I start with an explanation of the basics (What exactly is autism? And what is a GFCF diet, and how does it work?), information the parents need to have in detail, because starting the child on this diet is almost always the first step in treatment.

For many of my parents, this part of the initial consultation is merely reinforcing some things they already know—as I've said, these parents are, for the most part, people who've made themselves medically savvy. But autism can take so many forms, the symptoms can vary so widely, and the progress of the treatment is absolutely predicated upon how each child responds as an individual to each step along the way, so it's crucial that our communication be clear and thorough from the start. For a parent whose child may be medically homeless—who has likely endured more than one 5-minute audience with a pediatrician or neurologist or other specialist who has offered no real and practical solutions to their child's problems—this time can seem precious. It can feel like salve on a wound that has no scab, a long-infected wound that can now begin to heal.

WHAT IS AUTISM?

Imagine a landscape that was once lush with green foliage drying out and turning brown. The beds of creeks that once bubbled with life-giving water are emptying, and the trees and bushes on their former banks are leafless, nothing more really than sticks shriveled in brown, cracked dirt. Into this landscape come researchers—scientists who want to find out what has happened to this once-rich place. Why has it become a wasteland?

The researchers will immediately note that the annual rainfall in this place is well below average, that daily temperatures are scorching, and that harsh winds regularly blow through; some of the researchers will lay the blame for the land's regression on these observable facts.

Now, none of the researchers doubt that the wind and the rain and the sun had an impact on the land, but some of them won't be convinced that these are the only factors that contributed to the area's decline. After all, they will reason, this land has always faced hard weather conditions, and it was hardy enough to thrive at one time. What *changed?*

These unsatisfied researchers will dig a little deeper. They'll test the soil and find that it lacks the nutrients it needs to support life. They'll want to know where the nutrients have gone. They'll dig even deeper into the dirt, call for more and different tests, discover, perhaps, that there's an organism that's been introduced into the soil, greedily claiming for its own survival all the nutrients that used to go to the trees. Or perhaps they'll find there are toxins in the soil, industrial waste transported there on the currents of the now-dry creeks, and the trees won't grow because the land is now poisoned.

The point is that they won't be satisfied with explanations only their eyes can see. They'll want to know *why* they're seeing it. And what they will learn, in the end, is that what they can see—the leaf-less trees and the cracked creek beds—are only *symptoms* of a larger problem: the bacteria or the toxins that they couldn't see until they really dug for the answers.

So it is with autism.

You and I are part of an ever-expanding group of parents and clinicians who aren't satisfied that autism begins and ends with the blank, affectless looks on the faces of our children. We want to know what lies beyond those expressions—what has gone wrong at a deeper level that is causing the land to look so barren? In this book, we are going to embark on a sort of archeological dig, down to the depths of autism, to discover that the disease begins at the molecular level—and that it is at this molecular level, deep within the child's body, where the healing can also begin.

Three standard areas doctors currently look at to make a diagnosis of autism are lack of communication skills; lack of social skills, such as the inability to make eye contact; and the presence of atypical be-haviors such as stimming or tantrum throwing. When these three observable phenomena are present in a child, the diagnosis is autism. Dr. Sid Baker, a former associate professor at Yale Medical School who cofounded the Defeat Autism Now! movement, has il-lustrated this concept beautifully using the intersecting circles of the Venn diagram. (See figure 1.1.)

But wait. Let's dig a little deeper. And let's start our excavation with the work that Leo Kanner first shared with us in that seminal 1943 paper. Kanner's original studies of autism were focused around 11 children. In the studies of these children he notes about

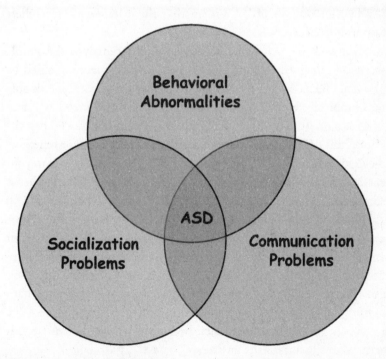

Figure 1.1   Courtesy of Sid Baker

Case #1, "Eating has always been a problem for him. He has never shown a normal appetite." Of Case #2, he observes that the child has "large and ragged tonsils." Of Case #3 he says, "Diarrhea and fever following smallpox vaccination . . . healthy except for large tonsils and adenoids."

In fact, in each of the 11 children he studied, Kanner found health issues severe enough to be remarked upon, from the child who nursed poorly and thus needed to be tube-fed for the first year of her life to the child who frequently required hospitalization for repeated colds, bronchitis, streptococcus infections, and impetigo. But as the definition of autism evolved over the decades since Kanner's original work, these physical signs got lost in the shuffle. Perhaps they were disregarded because the physical illnesses varied so greatly, each child manifesting illness in a different way or to a different degree, they were seen as peripheral to the all too obvious psychiatric components of autism that these long-ago researchers saw and described.

But what happens when we admit into our analysis the simple fact that a diagnosis of autism is almost invariably accompanied by physical illness? When we acknowledge that many autistic kids suffer chronically with colds and earaches, bronchitis, or other infections as a result of dysfunctional immune systems, or that 80 percent of our kids deal with the chronic diarrhea, constipation, or reflux indicative of a gut disease? Does a warning bell begin to sound in your ears? Are you thinking: *Hold on just a second here!* Maybe there's something going on outside the child's brain. Maybe this isn't all about a kid's brain being unable to direct him to produce age-appropriate behavior, or take part in age-appropriate social exchange, or enjoy the development of age-appropriate communication skills. Maybe, like those trees shriveling on a barren landscape, their growth stunted by bacteria and toxins, there is something that's *causing* this kid's brain to malfunction. Maybe that thing, like the tree's sick soil, is the child's sick body. Maybe we just can't see it until we really dig for the answers.

STATIC ENCEPHALOPATHY

Digging a little deeper, under the skin of a disease and beyond its observable signs and symptoms, is, of course, the obvious goal of medical research. The more we know about a disease, the better we are able to treat it. A fuller understanding of causes has historically led the medical establishment to revise outdated diagnoses and adopt more advanced treatment options. These revisions can come about because researchers discover, for example, a heretofore unknown neurotransmitter and its link to illness. Or because science provides us with a new or more accurate diagnostic tool. And revisions in medical thinking can come about because of cultural shifts, as a community absorbs and adapts to new scientific knowledge, technology, and social progress—and sometimes even because its tastes in fashion change.

Follow me through just one instance of a change in fashion that made us think a little differently about the human body. It used to be the conventional wisdom that we women were a weak lot, unable to withstand a great deal of physical activity without becoming winded, light-headed, and even swooning. We were a fragile sex, delicate creatures, vulnerable to *the vapors*. Or at least delicacy was attributed to upper-class women, those who had the luxury of domestic help and could afford to spend their days tightly laced into the whalebone corsets that sculpted their figures into fashionable hourglasses with wasp waists—and, in the process, squeezed and displaced their internal organs. Then Coco Chanel came along and created clothing that did away with those corsets. When kidneys, stomachs, and lungs were free to function within the whole, naturally shaped body cavity, well! Lo and behold! Along come Mia Hamm, Venus Williams, and Jackie Joyner-Kersee.

It was an unenlightened society that bound half its people in stays and laces for the sake of a rigid ideal of physical beauty and then declared that those who were so bound possessed naturally inferior physical temperaments. The connection between having one's internal organs strangled and becoming winded seems laughably obvious to us now. It was the same lack of enlightenment that, only 40 years ago, led society to label the moms of autistic kids *refrigerator mothers,* thought to be so cold, such unnatural nurturers, that they drove their children to mental illness.

While the term *refrigerator mom* has been discredited, we still hear the label *static encephalopathy* applied to autism. Static encephalopathy, this tongue twister term, means a disease of the brain that gets neither better nor worse. It means permanent brain damage. Fixed. Unchanging. Dead end. And there are still far too many pediatricians and neurologists and therapists who will use the term to refer to autistic patients. Still far too many who think of a diagnosis of autism as the first step on a path that leads only to institutionalization. Those doctors and therapists who use the term static encephalopathy to refer to the condition of an autistic child have stopped digging. They are the contemporary counterparts of the old-time physicians who insisted that females were innately fragile.

How do you find out if the doctor to whom you have entrusted the care of your autistic child is equipped to treat the disease progressively?

My advice is to ask the practitioner straight out, at your first appointment, if he or she believes autism is a static encephalopathy. If he or she answers yes—if he or she even pauses to consider the question or does anything other than recoil at the mere suggestion, run. Say, "Thank you very much for your time," and move as quickly as you can get your child's little feet to go out of there. A practitioner who doesn't know that recovery is possible—who hasn't read that it is scientifically plausible, who doesn't believe that in your child it is probable—will not be able to help your child recover. Now what about the practitioner who tells you that she doesn't know how to guide the process but is willing to be a part of a team that includes someone who does? Kiss that practitioner's whole face and make her an assistant coach. Then go home and boot up your computer and log on to one of the websites referenced in the Resources section of this book where you will find listings of biomedically trained autism specialists. Find the one nearest to you and schedule your child for the earliest available appointment.

Autism is a disease that impacts the entire family. Mom and Dad are physically drained from around-the-clock care giving, emotionally exhausted from trying to soothe unending screams and tantrums, and likely to be under severe marital stress because of it. The divorce rate among parents of autistic kids is so high that 80 percent of autistic kids grow up in single parent homes. Siblings can feel neglected or resentful because of the hours of attention and the amount of family funds that must be devoted to their sick brother or sister. Frequently, grandparents and other members of the extended family are drawn out of retirement and into the battered family unit to lend a hand. Everyone in our community tries to adopt my mother, who has come out of retirement to cook, run errands, and care for our family. Autism is a difficult diagnosis with a broad impact on everyone who loves the afflicted child; you do not need to exacerbate the stress by trusting the care of your sick kid to a doctor who doesn't understand that corsets have gone out of style.

THE NEW DEFINITION OF AUTISM

What you are looking for in the clinician who will treat your autistic child is someone who is willing to get his or her hands dirty—to dig with you deep into the "soil" that supports your child's health.

The old idea of autism relies on three overlapping areas of *observable* deficits—communication, socialization, and behavior—for its definition. Biomedical practitioners know that these three areas of deficit are only the *signs* of the disease. They are merely the ways we can see the disease manifested with our eyes. A true understanding of autism requires that we go much deeper within the body, to a *biochemical* level.

All right, don't panic; I've already told you I don't like biochemistry either. I'll make this as painless as possible. Biochemistry is, simply, the study of the chemistry of the living world. It's the study of the basic chemical compounds that all plants and animals use to sustain life. These compounds are created in every living creature at the cellular level, but biochemistry is not about cells; it goes even deeper. It's about the molecules that make up the cells and the atoms that make up the molecules; even the single-celled amoeba undergoes within its microscopic body life-sustaining processes that take place at a molecular level. Molecules of nourishment—things such as food and vitamins that are the specific sustenance of each different life form—are chemically changed into the compounds such as sugars or proteins that the species needs to stay alive.

Notice that in the last paragraph I said *processes*. Plural. The work of taking in, for example, vitamin D from a food source, or a vitamin supplement, or transdermally from the rays of the sun and transforming it chemically so that it can become one of the building blocks of a strong tooth or a toned muscle is repeated over and over and over again at the cellular level. At the same time, the work of taking in vitamin E from a food source or a vitamin supplement and transforming it into a compound the body needs is also going on, over and over and over, as is the work of taking in and transforming every other raw material the body needs to produce all the complex sugars and proteins, hormones, antioxidants, and neurotransmitters we need to make us our healthy, thriving human selves. Some of these processes are so important that they occur thousands and thousands of times inside every cell of your body every minute of every day.

I find that thinking of a cell as a gearbox inside of, say, a clock, is a good visual image to help in understanding these constant and complex interacting cycles of molecular transformation that go on within it. Picture this: inside your gearbox are dozens of individual gears, each one turning regularly and at a speed that allows it to mesh seamlessly with the gear next to it. This first seamless meshing allows the next gear to mesh with the gear next to it, and so on—all the dozens of gears working in harmony to keep the gearbox in motion, so when you check the time on the clock it's always accurate.

Seamless perpetual motion of the cellular gearbox is, of course, the ideal. But we all know what happens to an efficient network of gears when one of them gets gummed up by dirty oil or a piece of lint, or one of them gets wet and starts to rust, or one of them loses a tooth so it can't catch and connect with the gear next to it. One of the gears goes down, and none of the gears can make their revolutions as efficiently. The machine breaks down, right? At least until you can get the gears cleaned out and polished up and generally repaired.

What researchers have found, in studying the biochemistry of autistic kids, is that autism is a disease in which our kids' gearboxes—their cells—are gummed up. Rusty. Broken. The three main culprits in jamming up our kids' clockworks are chronic inflammation, oxidative stress, and toxicity. We'll talk about each of these three main culprits in more detail in a minute, but right now take a look at figure 1.2, again by Sid Baker, to help to fix the relationship of these big three clearly in your mind: where the three intersecting circles of inflammation, oxidative stress, and toxicity overlap in the Venn diagram, there is the new, true definition of autism.

Now what's fascinating about our new, true definition of autism is that there are researchers in many fields of medicine pursuing answers to "What caused it?" and "What will fix it?" for their disease of interest. And they are finding that the same big three culprits are at work in their diseases—chronic inflammation, oxidative stress, and toxicity. I suspect we will find over time that it is the genetic vulnerabilities of the individual in the face of these big three that give rise to whatever disease develops.

So autism is a series of malfunctioning—gummed up, rusty, broken—gears, or cycles, interacting in a child's body. These dysfunctional cycles play havoc with the child's cellular chemistry. His body is not able to correctly make or distribute the compounds needed by his anatomical systems—including the immune, digestive, and sulfur metabolism and detoxification systems—so that they can work efficiently. It's the dysfunction of these cellular cycles that

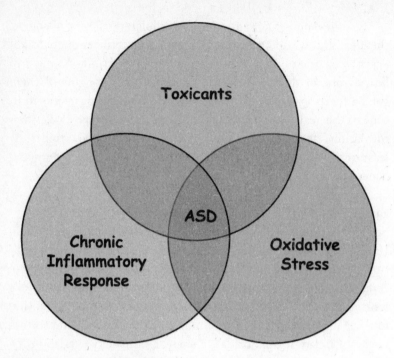

Figure 1.2   Courtesy of Sid Baker

causes the child to exhibit the eccentric behaviors that have been construed as the entirety of autism. When we fix the cycles, when we address *all* the issues that Kanner identified, an autistic child can recover his or her physical, and mental, health. When we get those clockwork gears cleaned out and meshing smoothly again, nourishment and nutrients can again be correctly processed by his systems and ultimately find their way to his brain, clearing the fog that has prevented him from fully experiencing the joys of life, learning, and loving.

THE BIG THREE: INFLAMMATION, OXIDATIVE STRESS, AND TOXICITY

So we know that it is inflammation, oxidative stress, and toxicity gumming up our kids' gearboxes. These are the three major biochemical problems our kids face. Let those processes go awry and it will manifest as the immune system disruption, the gut dysfunction, and the sulfur metabolism interruption that we see so commonly in our children. Let's look at each of these biochemical problems in a bit more depth so that we can understand exactly what we're talking about.

Chronic Inflammation

Inflammation is our body's natural biological response to infection or trauma; importantly, it's not a word that is interchangeable with infection. Infection is *caused* by pathogens, such as bacteria and viruses. Inflammation is the body's *response* to infection, or to other irritants such as splinters, broken bones, sprains, or bruises; it is the body healing itself by sending more plasma and white blood cells to the site of the offended tissue.

When you cut your finger instead of the next slice of cherry pie, your vascular system immediately rushes to your defense, directing blood to the site of the wound. This rush of blood is the beginning of *acute* inflammation, and without it, without your body sending its natural healing components to the site of the injury, that cut on your finger would never heal.

Chronic inflammation, however—the kind most autistic kids contend with—is when the inflammation is prolonged over an extended period of time. When this happens, inflammation stops being functional and becomes dysfunctional. It happens when your body recognizes an injury of some type as going on long enough for the type of cells in that specific tissue of the body to actually change their makeup and their normal responses to signals from other cells and molecules. This shift of cellular arrangement can readily be characterized as a war, the cells simultaneously and constantly both healing and destroying the tissue where they reside.

If your child is suffering from chronic diarrhea or chronic constipation, chances are it's because he's also suffering from chronic gut inflammation. Somewhere in his bowels or intestines or stomach lining, his body is at war with itself.

Oxidative Stress

Oxidative stress happens when there is an imbalance between the cellular production of reactive oxygen and a body's ability to rid itself of reactive oxygen.

What does *that* mean?

Within each cell of our body is a natural defense mechanism against charged particles called reactive oxygen species (ROS). ROS can be oxygen ions, peroxides, or unstable electrons, the *free radicals* we hear so much about in health news as well as in advertising copy for anti-aging cosmetics. ROS, however, are not entirely bad things. They are created as a by-product of the natural metabolism of oxygen, and they have a few important roles to play in our bodies, including enabling intracellular communication and signaling the immune system that there are foreign pathogens in the body that it must mobilize to attack and kill.

It is when there is an overproduction of ROS, coupled with a body's decreased capacity to naturally reduce the amount of ROS in its system, that oxidative stress sets in. This imbalance is a component of many diseases, including Parkinson's and Alzheimer's as well as autism. It means, simply, that the body can't cope with the amount of ROS it contains. The ROS begin to destroy cellular components such as proteins or DNA, or mitochondria, which are the cell's "power plants," generating most of the cell's chemical energy. An overabundance of ROS damages the structure of the cell and, in extreme cases, causes the cell to collapse and die.

One of the body's most effective natural defenses against excessive ROS is *glutathione*. Keep that word—glutathione—in the back of your mind for now; we'll talk much more about it as we move into our discussion of recovery.

Toxicity

The word *toxicity* has two meanings, both of which are important to understanding its role in autism.

The first meaning is *the quality or the condition of being toxic.* When I first explain this meaning to parents during their initial office visit, the near-universal response is a lengthy pause followed by a dropped jaw as they realize what I'm saying to them: Our kids are toxic! *Poisoned?*

Yes, they are. And, as you'll see, it's not only the parents of autistic kids who should be unnerved about how poisons are finding their way into our children's systems. No evil demon in a dirty black cloak is slithering silkily throughout the world, randomly slipping toxic spells and potions to our children while they sleep. The poisons are readily available at your friendly neighborhood grocery store. They are as present as the water we drink. They are as common as the air we breathe.

Say *what?*

Take a step back with me for a minute. A report issued by the Harvard Medical School's Center for Health and the Global Environment, "Inside the Greenhouse: The Impacts of CO_2 and Climate Change on Public Health in the Inner City," found that asthma among preschool children aged three to five years rose by 160 percent from 1980 to 1994. In the 20 years from 1975 to 1995, cancer rates rose for children by 20 percent, and one of the most rapidly increasing rates of cancer is in children under 13 years. The CDC and the AAP now concur with the alarming fact that one in six children have a developmental disorder or behavior problem—classified from ADD/ADHD (attention deficit hyperactivity disorder) to autism.

What's the coincidence? What other things are going on that might explain these crushing new trends? Again, it's parents—us ordinary folks—who are figuring out the answers well in advance of the curve: a 2008 Gallup poll found that up to 80 percent of respondents worried "a great deal" or "a fair amount" about polluted drinking water, soil contaminated by toxic waste, and air pollution.

Well, they should.

Persistent Organic Pollutants

The United Nations Environment Programme defines persistent organic pollutants (POPs) as "chemical substances that persist in the environment, bioaccumulate through the food web, and pose a risk of causing adverse effects to human health and the environment." But what exactly are POPs? Well, they are the more than 1,672,127,735 pounds of chemicals the Environmental Protection Agency (EPA) estimates are released into the environment each year. The 3,000 chemicals that are "approved" additives to the foods we eat. The approximately 1.2 billion pounds of pesticides sprayed annually on food and nonfood crops alike. And some of those pesticides are not merely a once-a-year insult to farmlands; they don't readily break down and can persist in the soil—and in the food that is grown in the soil—for generations.

POPs are the contents of common cleaning solvents. Pick up any one of the bottles or boxes you use regularly on cleaning day and you'll likely see some sort of warning prominently displayed on its back side. "Hazardous to humans and domestic animals." "Harmful if swallowed." "Use in well-ventilated room." "Avoid contact with skin and eyes. In case of contact, flush immediately and thoroughly with water for 15 minutes. Call a doctor or poison control center for more advice." These warnings are necessary—and often legally mandated—because your toilet bowl sanitizer and oven cleaner and silver polish are made with chemical compounds that have the potential, in large enough doses, to kill a healthy adult.

POPs are also heavy metals, such as lead, arsenic, cadmium, thallium, mercury, and 18 other chemical elements that have a measure of density at least five times that of water. These elements can enter the body by way of food, water, air, and absorption through the skin. Once in the body, they accumulate in layers of fat, competing with and displacing essential minerals such as calcium and zinc and disrupting normal organ function.

We have known for a long time about the dangers of these elements. The classic old play *Arsenic and Old Lace,* about two elderly spinsters who commit murder by lacing glasses of their homemade elderberry wine with arsenic, was written in 1939—but steps weren't taken to ban arsenic or thallium as ingredients for commercially available rat poison until 1984. Lead is so deadly that ages ago we discontinued its use in things such as plumbing fixtures, gasoline, and paint; we need look back no further than 2007 for a refresher course in its danger, to the devastation wrought upon so many families who unwittingly purchased toys made in China with lead paint. In 1992, the EPA issued a "Hazard Summary" that concluded that the cadmium released into the air we breathe through burning fossil fuels and municipal waste caused pulmonary irritation and kidney disease and was known to be a "developmental toxicant in animals, resulting in fetal malformations and other effects." Incredibly, however, the report completely ignored the simple fact that people share enough in common biochemically with every other animal on the planet that we routinely infer human toxicity from animal research; the EPA's report stated that "no conclusive evidence exists in humans."

As for mercury, the expression "mad as a hatter" comes to us from seventeenth-century France, where mercury poisoning was common among the hatmakers who used mercuric nitrate to soak hides and soften the skins.

How mercury gets into our bodies today is a bit more complex—and insidious. Let's start with electricity. Most of the world's electricity is produced by burning coal; in the United States alone, 54 percent of the electricity is produced from coal. It's likely that the power plant that delivers the juice to run your toaster and microwave and washing machine uses coal as its feedstock.

When coal is burned, it releases a number of pollutants into the atmosphere—ash, sulfur, and mercury. The mercury settles in bodies of water, or on land masses where it is eventually flushed into bodies of water. There, it's converted by microorganisms into methylmercury and eaten by sea life. Humans, in turn, eat the sea life—shrimp and salmon and tuna—who have eaten the mercury. It's not uncommon that, the morning after you've enjoyed that delicious, ginger-marinated tuna steak dinner, your mercury levels will have risen high enough for you to be considered mercury toxic.

Oil refineries, the improper disposal of old thermometers, the silver-colored amalgams that dentists routinely use to fill the cavities in your mouth—these are all sources of the mercury that ends up stored in human tissues. It is critical to the understanding of "heavy metal poisoning" that we take all these sources into account. Toxins are pervasive in our modern world, and the opportunity to be exposed to them is constant as we innocently go about our everyday lives. No one source is solely responsible for the rise of any disease, from asthma to cancer to autism. But I also have to say—because I promised to sidestep controversy only where I could—that mercury is commonly delivered directly into human bloodstreams by purposeful, medically approved, and usually governmentally mandated injection. It has been a component of childhood vaccinations since 1934—probably not coincidentally, just a few years before Kanner first described the then-emerging phenomenon of autism. Mercury, when it is used in an industrial setting, must be treated as a hazardous substance. The coal industry is under siege to retrofit its power plants with the technology that has the potential to remove over 90 percent of mercury emissions. Dentists, when removing mercury fillings from your mouth, must dispose of them as hazardous waste. Does it make any sense to you that a substance your dentist must dispose of in a red caution container *after* it is out of your mouth is any less toxic than when it is *in* your mouth? Blood levels as low as 19 µg/L are considered potentially toxic in adults; how did it become general practice to put 25 µg of the stuff into a syringe and pump up to four syringefuls at a time into a baby's body?

In addition to mercury, other POPs include free radicals. They are the unstable electrons inside our cells that destroy the cell structure and result in oxidative stress, and they are not created just by the natural metabolism of oxygen. Free radicals result from the toxins in pollutants such as cigarette smoke, coal-fired power plant emissions, alcohol, and radiation, and from the use of chemicals in foods and pesticides to grow our food. They also result from every pressure exerted on the human body—everything from the current condition of our once-pristine planet to problems that seem so much more immediate to our everyday lives, such as job pressures, deadlines, the financial markets. Free radicals result from the straightforward stress of day-to-day living. Stress, in families with autistic kids, includes the day-to-day management of their child's disease, so you can see why I often recommend dietary changes and nutritional supplements for Mom and Dad too. A diet of whole foods supplemented with vitamins and minerals will do even the healthiest among us a world of good, of course. That's because the effect of POPs is a problem that impacts every one of us. But how can we measure that impact?

According to Lynn Goldman, a pediatrician and epidemiologist at Johns Hopkins University, "Concern is growing worldwide over the long term health effects of chemicals known as persistent organic pollutants. Exposure to POPs is shifting the IQ of the population downward—more developmentally-challenged people and fewer gifted people." One measure might be, then, to compare the change in IQ scores. James Flynn, Emeritus Professor at the University of Otego in Dunedin, New Zealand, and renowned intelligence researcher, found and published results in February 2009 that the average IQ of 14 year olds declined from 1980 to 2008—the first such decline since the test was developed in 1912.

Researchers from the Mount Sinai School of Medicine in New York put a dollar value on lower IQs in a 2006 report, "Mental

Retardation and Prenatal Methylmercury Toxicity." Using national blood mercury data from the CDC, these researchers found that between 316,588 and 637,233 children each year have blood mercury levels associated with the loss of IQ points. "The resulting loss of intelligence caused diminished economic productivity that persists over the lifetime of these children." The cost of this diminished productivity from mercury sources alone? The researchers estimated it at $8.7 billion annually and concluded, "This significant toll threatens the economic health and security of the United States and should be considered in the debate on mercury pollution controls."

What does this annual $8.7 billion translate to for an afflicted child? The researchers estimated that each IQ point lost was worth between $15,000 and $25,000 in wages the child will never be able to earn.

One study that measures the horrible vulnerability of human health to POPs as they relate specifically to autism was completed in 2006 by scientists at the University of Texas Health Science Center in San Antonio, Texas. This study, "Environmental mercury release, special education rates, and autism disorder: an ecological study of Texas," shows a statistically significant link between pounds of industrial release of mercury and increased autism rates. It shows as well—and, for the first time, in a riveting, graphic manner—a statistically significant association between proximity to a source of mercury release and increased risk of autism.

In setting out to determine whether the proximity to sources of environmental mercury release was a predictor of autism prevalence, the authors observed rates of autism in 1,040 Texas school districts for 1990–1993, and again for 1998–2000. They then compared these rates to the toxic release inventory (TRI) reported by 39 coal-fired power plants and 56 industrial facilities in the state of Texas. What they found was a near overlap of statistics—when the results are expressed as darker and lighter areas on a map of Texas, the reported increases in pollution created a near-exact overlay of the increases in cases of autism. According to the report, "On average, for each 1000 pounds of environmentally released mercury, there was . . . a 61% increase in the rate of autism."

"The effects of persistent, low-dose exposure to mercury pollution, in addition to fish consumption, deserves attention," Dr. Raymond T. Palmer, the study's lead author, has reported.

I'll say.

While we cannot consider mercury, whether delivered into a child's system through power plant emissions or vaccinations or dental fillings, as the lone factor contributing to the rise of autism rates—if we do, then we are putting our heads in the sand about the enormity of the problem and the nuances of the cumulative effects of prolonged toxic exposure—we can use mercury in yet another example of the ubiquity of environmental toxicants.

In January 2009, a new study was published by the Institute for Agriculture and Trade Policy that found mercury in the high-fructose corn syrup (HFCS) that is commonly used to sweeten everything from the breads and cereals, to the soups, condiments, lunch meats, and candy bars that are almost universally on our grocer's shelves—and in our homes. The path of the mercury contamination was fairly direct: caustic soda is used in the manufacture of HFCS; mercury can be used to manufacture caustic soda. In 15 of the 55 brand-name food products analyzed in these tests, the food processors—likely unthinkingly—had used caustic soda that had been manufactured using the mercury process.

"Mercury is toxic in all its forms. Given how much high fructose corn syrup is consumed by children"—12 to nearly 100 teaspoons a day, on average—"it could be a significant additional source of mercury never before considered," said Dr. David Wallinga, a coauthor of the study.

When you are confronted by a claim that any one suspicious environmental toxin, or source of toxin, has been "definitively" ruled out as a cause of disease, remember this: it is unlikely that it is *one* mercury-tainted bowl of cereal, or *one* day of breathing oil refinery emissions, or *one* vaccination shot that is causing the epidemic of disease we face today; it is the cumulative effects of prolonged exposure to myriad poisons.

The POPs we've just talked about are merely a sampling of the sort of pollutants that have altered our earth's environment and made it less healthful. But the POP label doesn't include other equally problematic environmental problems we humans have created for ourselves. Take antibiotics, for instance.

It's unlikely you'll run into any doctor who would deny the obvious benefits of having antibiotics in our disease-fighting toolbox. They can be lifesaving when used appropriately. But their *over*use—in humans, and in the animals humans consume as food—is another part of what Maureen McDonnell, a brilliant nurse I know, calls "the big experiment we have been conducting on the human race since the end of World War II." At that time, coal burning increased in tandem with the rise in global population and all the new people in the world who needed heat and light, we first began the widespread attempt to control disease through vaccination programs, and antibiotics first became available for use by the general population.

Antibiotics, in the course of doing their work killing off bad bacteria, also kill off good bacteria—or what are called *probiotics*. The reduction of probiotics in a human gut can lead to the overgrowth of other bacteria that don't normally live in our gut—a phenomenon we call dysbiosis. These interloping bacteria can, in turn, produce *endotoxins*. Endotoxins are poisons that are present in the cell walls of some of these bacteria and that are released only after the bacteria have died. Among their ill effects are fever, chills, shock, and increased permeability—or *leakage*—in capillaries and other membranes. A prolonged presence of endotoxins in a person's system can cause excessive fermentation in the gut, which leads to the creation of ever more and derivative toxins—and an even greater toll on the digestive tract, until it leaks like a sieve. They can, further, trigger sensitivity to certain foods in the compromised digestive system, weaken the immune system (70 percent of which is located along our digestive tract), and overwhelm the liver, an organ that is charged with expelling toxins from the human body.

Yet, despite all these potential ill effects, practitioners in the Defeat Autism Now! movement use antibiotics when they are necessary. As I said, they can be lifesaving. But we use them judiciously, and balance their use by giving the patient supplemental probiotics so that her system can maintain its fair share of good bacteria. To paraphrase a lyric by the famous songwriter Sting: "Miracles of science so often go from a blessing to a curse." Antibiotics are, without question, a miracle of science; the challenge is to use them wisely, to benefit human health, so that the good they are quite capable of doing doesn't turn into something bad . . . and, then, into something even worse.

MALNUTRITION AND AUTISM

I'm deliberately using a word that, to the great many of us, evokes what happens only in developing countries in the midst of famine: malnutrition. The effects of severe malnutrition—the distended bellies below rib cages in achingly sharp relief—move those of us in the developed world to, simultaneously, disbelief and gratitude. Disbelief that we as a world community have not yet found a way to provide enough food to all our people, and gratitude for what we *are* able to provide to our own children. Unlike most parents in the developed world today, however, I am deeply, sadly, fiercely aware of how shaky the nutritional foundation is for even children in the developed world—the children you and I tuck into bed every night between clean sheets, kissing their freshly scrubbed faces, laying them down to sleep with what we think of as well-fed bellies.

The hard, stark fact is that many of the foods readily available to us today in our supermarkets are, to put it mildly, less than valuable, nutritionally. They have been stripped of so many of the elements that are essential to sustain life that we call them "junk food." Just as when we put a lower-grade gasoline in our car it can cause engine knocks or decreased gas mileage, when we fuel our bodies with junk, we can't expect peak performances from them. What is often sur- prising—even shocking—is the wide range of foods that can be classified as junk.

Foods that have been stripped of their indispensable vitamins, minerals, and fiber are called *denatured*. They reach this ominous state in several ways. Let's start with packaged, processed foods— the lunch meats and cereals and breads most kids are used to eating for breakfast and finding in their lunch boxes. The manufacturers of this food remove healthy elements from their raw materials—no- tably the bran, or fiber, from flours—to make these foods "kid friendly." At the same time, they add preservatives or manipulate natural components of food, like their oils, to preserve shelf life and make the food convenient for busy moms and dads. When a parent becomes aware of just how developmentally *unfriendly* these foods are for their kids—as well as just how much strain they place even on the healthiest adult system by depriving it of essential nutri- tion—the parent can certainly seek out alternative foods for the family: foods that are grown organically and, ideally, locally, and left whole. These alternatives, however, often make a bigger dent in the family food budget than their junk counterparts and, for some fam- ilies, are simply unaffordable. We are not talking here about luxury food items—we are talking about apples and carrots and spinach. We have clearly reached a food crisis when it is cheaper to buy in- dustrially grown, nutrient-depleted canned green beans than it is to buy fresh, in season ones from the farmer in the next county.

The blame for this inequity can be laid largely at the door of the large industrial farms that dominate our food network, where the bulk of our contemporary food supply is grown. Through agricultural prac- tices that revolve around corporate profits rather than human health—such as the use of convenient and cheap but deadly chemical pesticides—the foods they grow, and that we eat, are simply less nourishing than the foods that were available to previous generations.

Take, for example, spinach—maybe Popeye's favorite, but likely not as popular with the toddler set. "Take just one bite," I remember my mother begging me when I was a child and the hated vegetable turned up on the family dinner table. Well, just one bite of the spinach my mother insisted I eat in 1965 would have contained nearly five times the amount of vitamin C my own kids will get today, if I can cajole them to eat a same-sized bite. For comparison, 100 g of spinach in 1950 contained 150 mg of vitamin C; in 1963, the same amount contained 100 mg. In 1982, 100 g of spinach contained 63 mg of vitamin C and, by 1994, it contained just 13 mg.

Calcium, phosphorous, B_{12} ... choose your nutrient, none of them are as abundantly available in the spinach or carrots or apples we eat today as once they were. Heart disease, Alzheimer's, autism ... pick your disease; all these conditions are exacerbated because people are simply not getting the nutrition human bodies need to stay healthy and fight disease. Denatured foods likely have some part in even the contemporary obesity epidemic. Follow the logic: we have to eat nearly five times the amount of spinach today to receive the same nutritional value our parents and grandparents enjoyed in one serving. But our bodies still crave the nutrients they need to work efficiently. If a body doesn't get the proper vitamins and minerals it needs, it will continue to crave food in greater and greater quantities in its quest to satisfy its needs and stay alive.

It's not just plant foods that have been stripped of their nutritional values. Neither meat nor dairy products are as nourishing to us as once they were. Think about it: livestock is fed a diet of grain that, in most cases, is itself grown in depleted soil; if we feed cows and chickens and pigs a diet of denatured food, depriving them of vital nutritional elements, how could it be possible that their sickly meat is nourishing to us?

We humans are very clever. We've set up a food network for ourselves that is starving us. Depriving our cells of the essential raw materials they need to build strong bones and muscle. Destroying our bodies from the inside out. Combine a severely polluted environment with across-the-board nutritional deficiencies and you get across-the-board weakened bodies—even if the weakening occurs in ways too subtle for a strong adult or conventionally healthy youngster to notice on a day-to-day basis. It should come as little surprise, then, that we have created for ourselves an epidemic of poorly nourished, toxic children.

We have created the epidemic of ASD.

As we consider ASDs, it should be intuitive for us to understand that depending on the individual, on the "doses" of toxins, and on the timing of those "doses" there will be a tremendous variation in how those toxins impact any single human body. We call that a spectrum. And as we increasingly understand that autism is a broad spectrum of disease, we understand that ADD, learning disabilities, and oppositional defiance, along with PDD and Asperger's, are all variations on the autism theme.

THE GENETIC FACTOR

"To cling to a purely genetic explanation for autism is a desperate attempt to maintain the illusion that one lives in a comfortable and rational world where new chemicals and technologies always mean progress; experts are always objective and thorough; corporations are honest; and authorities can be trusted. That human actions, rather than genes, might be responsible for compromising the health of a significant portion of a whole generation is so painful as to be, for many, unthinkable."

Martha Hebert, MD, PhD
Harvard Medical School

I'm betting on your next question: If the environment we've created is such a dangerous place for our children, why aren't even more children diagnosed with ASDs? Why aren't *all* children sick? This is where the second meaning of toxicity comes in. Toxicity also refers to *the degree to which a particular substance can cause harm to an organism.* One of the central concepts of toxicity is that it is *dose dependent.*

Let's look at a well-known, if fairly creepy, toxin to understand dose dependency: snake venom. If you are bitten on the foot by a rattlesnake, whether that bite is fatal is determined by how much of the venom gets into your system and how quickly it is allowed to flow through your bloodstream. If you receive first aid rapidly, keep your foot below the heart, and perhaps—with much difficulty—remain calm and immobile so that your excited heart and muscles don't pump the venom quite as fast throughout your body, you have a good chance of surviving. A small amount of the venom won't cause as much damage to your systems as will a larger amount. In other words, the dose makes the poison.

Whether a child will develop autism is dependent on how exposed he is to a toxic environment. It will depend on how well her systems are nourished and can effectively battle back against the environmental toxins to which she is exposed. And it will depend on whether he is genetically predisposed to contract disease.

GENETIC PREDISPOSITIONS

Sometimes, my patients' parents will wonder why the "family history" section of my first visit with their child takes so long and is so detailed. They know that if Grandma had diabetes, they should be watched for the signs of diabetes developing in them as well. Same for heart disease, stroke, and other diseases. But they are confused about my questions about diseases such as Alzheimer's or adult-onset schizophrenia. There is often no history of autism in their family and, because I've usually just explained to them that autism is a contemporary epidemic, they wonder why I'm looking for a generational history of illness to relate to it.

I'm not.

Not in the conventional sense of saying that because a patient's mother was diagnosed with breast cancer at a certain age, the patient has to be monitored for it too, and well before that same age.

No. What I'm looking for is a history of disease that will give me a clue as to what organ systems are historically more likely to be vulnerable to the modern-day onslaught of toxic exposure. How well her body is going to be able to deal with a toxic assault based on how well other members of her family have fared in a steadily worsening global environment. Does Grandpa have Alzheimer's? Does Dad suffer from reflux? Does Mom's family tend to develop autoimmune disease? Does the sibling of a purely autistic child present with ADHD?

Remember that autism is a spectrum disease. It manifests itself in a maddening variety of physical illnesses. If a person is full grown, 30 years old, and in generally good health, the ill effects of environmental toxins are going to manifest in that person in ways that are different from how the same toxins, in the same amounts, will impact a five-year-old with systems that are not as big or heavy, nor yet fully developed. If a person is 60 years old, and has started to let her health decline, the toxins will impact her differently from the way they impact the 60-year-old who eats a diet rich in fruits and vegetables and plays a mean match or two of tennis three mornings a week. I want to find out how well the child's family has fared in the past, how much toxic insult they were or were not able to tolerate. *How* were they able to deal with it? At what age did the insult exceed what their body was able to take, and how was the disease process manifested in them?

I want to find these things out—and here is the hardest part of all the things I have to tell you in this book—because we have created such a toxic world that it is not a matter of *whether* a person will be stricken with a disease, but a matter of *which* disease will strike and how intensely it will manifest itself.

"Which disease" and "how intensely" are fundamentally a part of how each individual is genetically programmed.

Let's talk about tobacco again. Why isn't every smoker dying of cancer? Why did my neighbor's 17-year-old son, who started smoking only two years ago, die of lung cancer last month, but your Aunt Mamie just celebrated her eighty-seventh birthday, and she's been puffing down two packs a day since 1945?

Environment, diet, and general good health, as well as genetics, have all very probably figured into the equation. A child who is diagnosed with ASD will very probably have some degree of disadvantage in all these areas. The insult will exceed what his body is individually able to cope with. The disease process will manifest itself sooner, with a lower cumulative dose of toxin, and cause more significant illness, than in the next person. Our children are the canaries in the coal mine.

Think of your child's body as a cup—a beautiful, fragile piece of translucent porcelain made not from clay and quartz and ash but from Mom and Dad's love and blood, chromosomes, and DNA. Into this beautiful, fragile cup are sometimes trickled, and too often poured, full force and sloshing, toxins of all types, day after day after day . . . The cup becomes discolored by the toxins, its shiny surface dulled, its delicate bowl cracked from the pressure of trying to contain the onslaught. His cup runneth over, so to speak, and it's our job to stop the gusher, level off the cup, and clean up the mess.

"MENTAL" PROBLEMS

A question parents ask me at our first meeting, almost to a person, is, why do the symptoms of autism present themselves as what appear to be *mental* problems? Let's go back to something I touched on in the last section to lead us to this answer; that is, the effects of a toxin are, in most cases, going to be more dramatic in a system that is less mature and, thus, still unable to fully defend itself against the attack. The rising rates of preschoolers with asthma and childhood cancer, as well as the rise in cases of autism, are evidence that we're asking our children to tolerate unprecedented amounts of toxins that the body is not designed to accommodate. One of the systems that is still developing in the child is his *brain*.

"We suspect low-dose exposure to various environmental toxicants, including mercury, occur during critical windows of neural development among genetically susceptible children and increase the risk for developmental disorders such as autism," the authors of the Texas study wrote in their report.

Exactly.

A young brain is essentially a construction zone, growing cells and developing neural pathways and undergoing myelination. Myelination is the process of a brain developing "white matter"— the fatty tissue that surrounds the more familiar "gray matter" and acts rather like the rubber casing around an electrical cord, grounding and directing the flow of electricity. In the case of the brain, the myelin grounds and directs the electrical impulses that are thought and emotion, learning and memory.

How long does this growth process of the brain take? How many years? Researchers have recently found, through the use of brain-imaging technologies, that a human brain remains a construction zone *until a person is in his early 20s.* And which is the last part of the brain to finish construction, around about when the child, now a young adult, is 22? The prefrontal cortex, where the capacity for critical thought and judgment reside.

When you are in an actual construction zone—building, for instance, a house—if you lay the foundation incorrectly or haphazardly, you will have trouble later with the alignment of the joists and the windows and the floorboards. So it is when the foundation of a young brain is compromised at the start of construction—later on, there will be trouble with language and behavior and motor skills.

Even more to the point, the brain is not, of course, built with concrete and drywall. It is built with fat. Mostly fat. Sixty percent of the brain's dry weight is fat.

Do you remember where I said toxic accumulations are stored in the body?

Right. In the fat.

Knowing that in the very years a child's brain is being built there is an ever-increasing chance that poison is mixed into the construction materials ought to terrify us.

RAPID RESPONSE

Now we're really getting right to the heart of the matter, right to what ASDs really are: *the neurological and biological expression of the impact of environmental toxins on genetically susceptible kids.* However shocking the existing medical establishment finds that definition, that's what autism is. Armed with the correct definition of the disease, doctors and medical researchers can properly investigate it and prescribe treatment. And let's keep in mind what it is we're prescribing treatment for: poison. Poison and its effects on the body.

Remember our creepy example, snake venom? No one would argue with you if you were bitten by a snake and you wanted treatment for it on the spot—if you tried to keep the venom from circulating in your bloodstream and reaching your organs where it does its damage, and you demanded the antidote to counter the poison's effects. Or how about this even more horrific example that might hit even closer to home: What if your toddler broke the child lock on the cabinet under the kitchen sink and took a swallow of Lime-A-Way? No one at the poison control center is going to put you on hold—they're going to give you instructions for treatment and they're going to give them to you *fast*. I have a friend who rushed her dog to the vet when he accidentally got into the part of the yard she'd just sprayed with weed killer and she saw him licking his paws. Different poisons can mean different problems—some shut down the nervous system, others will paralyze muscles, and still others attack the body in wholly different ways, but when they get inside living tissue, all poisons equal *emergency*. We all know they can cause long-term and permanent damage, and even death, if they remain unchecked in the bloodstream.

The toxins that are in our children's bodies, causing them to manifest the signs of autism, demand no less a rapid response than a snakebite or an accidental drink of cleaning fluid. They just haven't, up until recently, been able to get it.

WHERE RECOVERY LIES

When I go into my office in the morning and see a new patient listed on my daily appointment calendar, I always say a short but intense prayer before I let myself look at my electronic chart for the child's birth date, before I find out how old she is: Dear God, give me a nice, juicy two-year-old, a child who is just beginning to demonstrate the tell-tale signs of autism, a kid who hasn't been suffering for years and whose systems haven't been compromised, maybe irreparably, by prolonged exposure to poison.

Sometimes my prayer is answered. It's an innocent preschooler with his anxious parents coming through my office door. I rejoice because we've caught this one early, before his body has had years to be ill and sustain chronic damage. I know it will be a matter of only months—maybe even only weeks—before he begins to show signs of improvement and starts on his return journey to health.

Often, sadly, my new patients are older—four or five years old, or more. Maybe his parents were, like I was, reluctant to accept their child's diagnosis. Or maybe they spent months bumping up against brick walls—doctors who offered no hope, insistent that there was no treatment—until, at last, they heard about biomedical intervention through the Internet, or from a fellow parent who also has an autistic child, and they rushed to find a biomedical practitioner, only to bump up against a three-year waiting list. Or, perhaps, like

Angie's mother, for years they put their faith in the only medically accepted and prescribed solution—endless therapy—and finally just got scared enough to do something that is, unfortunately, still considered desperate by the powers that currently be. Ten-year-olds, like Angie, are some of my most difficult cases. They have been carrying around toxins in their systems for years. The treatment team—the parents, my staff, and I—have to roll our sleeves up above our elbows and get down to some hard work, hard work we are never sure, at that point, after years of toxic damage, can wholly restore the child's ability to achieve the full potential that God intended for her.

Let me be very clear at this juncture about several critical points:

1. The earlier a child begins treatment, preferably as soon as the first sign of autism is noticed, the easier treatment can be, and the more rapid the recovery.

2. Though the treatment will likely be more intense, and the intensity of a longer duration for an older child, these children can still recover, though the recovery may, in some cases, be only partial.

3. There is a definite progression to the steps of biomedical recovery for autistic children. Many of my patients' parents anticipate, as you might now be anticipating yourself, biomedical intervention focused on removing heavy metals from their child's system and are disappointed when I don't immediately begin their child on a specific chelation therapy—therapy that removes these toxins from the body. There is a good reason for the wait. In order for a child to successfully eliminate these toxins, we must first strengthen and support his body. Be patient. There are a myriad of ways to detoxify the body of heavy metals and other toxins; chelation is but one of them. Strong and supported with proper nutrition, following the steps I will

outline, your child will detoxify more readily than if we get the cart in front of the horse.

In order to fully understand the cumulative effects of environmental toxins in a child's body over a prolonged period of time, I want you to once again think of a gearbox. Think of dozens of gummed-up, rusty, broken gears but, this time, when you think of the clockwork, imagine a cartoon-style contraption run amok—the damaged gears spinning out of control, sliding against each other, popping out of alignment, careening into and connecting with any other old gear that happens to be nearby, whirling faster and faster and faster . . .

Smaller doses of environmental toxins that leak into the body slowly aren't usually as efficiently lethal as a large dose of snake venom or cleaning fluids. They are more insidious. They don't cause the body to shut down and stop working and abruptly die. No. They cause the body to—at a cellular level—spin out of control.

Take a look at figure 2.1. You'll see four sets of arrows arranged to form four different circular patterns; this concept and its illustration are borrowed from two brilliant clinicians and teachers, Dr. Elizabeth Mumper and Dr. Sidney Baker. Each one of these circular patterns represents one of the ways—one of the *vicious cycles*—in which an autistic child's physical systems are spinning out of control.

The first vicious cycle starts when the child's body is assaulted by an overload of environmental toxins—mercury, food additives, cleaning chemicals, and the like. Her body tries to detoxify itself. But, because of genetic susceptibility, malnourishment, continued exposure to toxins, or the injection of an extremely large amount of toxin directly into her body by way of multiple childhood vaccinations given at a single well child visit—or, most probably, a combination of these factors—her body is unable to detoxify itself as efficiently as the assault demands.

Then, because her body is not ridding itself of the poisons, they stay in place, stuck in her body, continuing to do their damage, interfering with her cells' ability to absorb minerals, vitamins, and

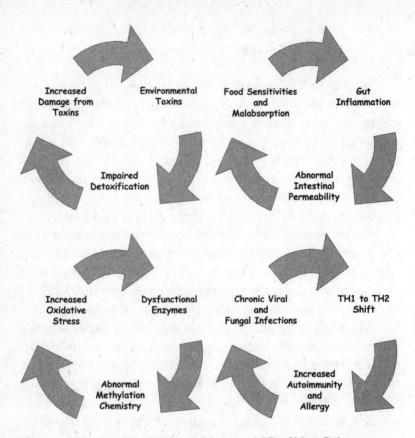

Figure 2.1 Courtesy of Dr. Elizabeth Mumper and Dr. Sidney Baker

other nutrients, blocking neurotransmitters, and generally wreaking havoc. If the cycle is not broken by intervention to improve her environmental conditions and support her body in its efforts to detoxify, it simply starts all over again, and with each vicious revolution, more damage is done.

The same phenomenon occurs in each of the other three cycles, like a snake eating its tail, except that these snakes interact, tangle together, intertwine, and end up in a knot that must be loosened and then untied before the child can recover. Through research and experience, biomedical practitioners know which part of the knot to begin untying first. And it's usually a different sequence with each child.

We're going to talk about each of these cycles, and how to break them, as we move into our discussion of treatment. Right now, I want to direct your attention to figure 2.2, the last of Sid Baker's Venn diagrams. With beautiful simplicity, it explains how we are going to treat your child's autism by repairing her damaged biochemical pathology. Within that balance, where Sid Baker's circles overlap, there lies the key to recovery. We are going to help her body to detoxify itself. We are going to provide her with anti-inflammatory agents of many sorts to reduce her chronic inflammation and repair

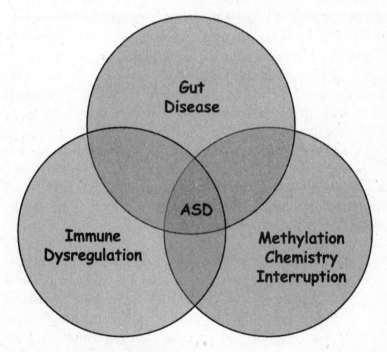

Figure 2.2   Courtesy of Sid Baker

its damage. We are going to supplement her with antioxidants to keep her cells from sustaining structural damage. Each individual child will need more or less help in each of these areas, and we are going to work to find the balance that your individual child requires. We will make these interventions in the context of bowel disease, immune dysfunction, and methylation chemistry support, again in a balance that your child requires.

THE ROLE OF NUTRITION IN TREATING ASD

Now we know where recovery lies. Where does it begin? Which cycle do we ungum and polish and fix first?

The human body comes equipped with an incredible, built-in defense system. But when the toxic burden the body must bear exceeds the body's ability to manage those toxins—that is, when the nutritional needs to manage those toxins exceeds the nutrient supply the body can deliver to the bloodstream; when the toxic burden challenges the efficient use of the nutrients the body is receiving—it can no longer function as it was designed to do. The first step in recovery is, therefore, to improve the quality of the child's nutritional status so that his body's natural, built-in defense system can begin to heal and start to work as it's supposed to.

One medical wit once tweaked an old adage to come up with the saying "The road to good health is paved with good intestines." But why is the gastrointestinal (GI) tract so important? Here are the five very good reasons why the GI tract is critical to our autistic kids.

1. The GI tract is one of the body's physical barriers protecting it and defending it against bacteria, viruses, and other invasive substances such as xenobiotics. Xenobiotics are any chemicals that are found in a living organism that are foreign to its system. Antibiotics, for example, are xenobiotics because they are not manufac-

tured by the biological system itself. The word *xenobiotics,* more commonly, refers to environmental pollutants. Go back to our original football analogy for a minute—the gut is the defensive line that makes sure the opposition players who would invade your turf and defeat you don't get a chance to do it.

2. I've said this before, but it bears repeating: the largest part of the human immune system—a full 70 percent of it—is snuggled up next to and intimately associated with the gut wall. Strengthening and healing the gut has the ripple effect of starting to help the child's overtaxed immune system to normalize as well.

3. The vitamins and minerals processed in the gut for use by every other system and cell in the body are the critical cofactors for producing enzymatic reactions and managing metabolism. Think of the football analogy again. You can have all the trained players you need outfitted in the most sophisticated sports gear available, standing ready on a meticulously groomed field, but if you don't have an actual football handy, you don't have a game. Same with enzymes—they are the catalyst for every chemical reaction the body wants and needs to perform. Feed the child right and she will start to more efficiently produce the enzymes she needs to kick off every other biochemical process that needs to take place within her body.

4. Nutrients are precursors for neurotransmitters. Neurotransmitters are the chemicals that relay information from one area of the brain to another—they are the signals the brain, the quarterback, sends to enable all the other players on the team to rally as a coordinated fighting unit. If we improve the quality of the nutrients that are available to the child's body, we improve the quality and quantity of the neurotransmitters his body is able to produce—and, so, the quality and quantity of his brain performance.

5.　Serotonin is just one of the neurotransmitters the brain uses to communicate, but it is unique in that a full 90 percent of it is made by the digestive tract. Because of the widespread distribution of serotonin within the body, it influences either directly or indirectly approximately 40 million brain cells, including brain cells related to appetite and sleep, mood and memory, and learning and social behavior. It also influences a myriad of cell functions outside the brain. Fix the gut and you begin to normalize the child's serotonin level so that she is naturally more cheerful, less prone to tantrums, and more apt to sleep through the night—and if she starts to sleep through the night, so can her parents.

SIGNS AND SYMPTOMS OF GI PROBLEMS

Very simply, the health of the GI system is key in determining how well the body and the brain are able to function. Dr. Arthur Krigsman, a board-certified pediatric gastroenterologist with Thoughtful House Center for Children in Austin, Texas, is among the leaders in cataloging, evaluating, and treating the GI pathology of children with ASDs. Dr. Krigsman speaks modestly at conferences and when meeting with patients about the connection between gut and brain health, explaining that "whether treatment of the bowel disease is correlated with improvement in cognitive function is the subject of current research at Thoughtful House." He goes on to add, "At the very least, it is simply intuitive that a child who feels good will have greater benefit from the myriad of available behavioral interventions than the child who is experiencing flatulence, diarrhea, urgency, and abdominal pain."

Again, it is a matter of basic human compassion to offer a physically sick child relief from pain, whether or not you believe those physical symptoms are in any way associated with his perceived mental problems. But I want to ask you a straightforward, common-sense question: Is it possible for you to dismiss, as many clinicians infuriatingly continue to do, chronic diarrhea as a behavioral problem? Is it in any way rational to you that your child has *decided* to have watery, explosive stools, or has *decided* to retain gas so that her stomach bloats in grotesque mimicry of pregnancy? Dr. Krigsman reports that many of his patients' parents have said to him, as many of mine have said to me, "My child has never had a formed stool, ever." He has documented, through endoscopy, the enlarged lymph nodes, the gastric ulcerations, the inflammatory polyps, and the otherwise generally unhealthy colons common among ASD children. It is not within my ability to imagine enlarged lymph nodes, gastric ulcerations, or inflammatory polyps resulting from the willfulness of your average two-year-old.

The signs and symptoms of bowel problems are myriad. As you start your child on the GFCF diet that is the first step of biomedical intervention for autism, you and your practitioner will want to document the particular signs and symptoms your child is manifesting. They could be one or more of the following:

- chronic diarrhea or chronic constipation
- presence of blood, food, or mucus in stools
- foul-smelling stools
- stools of abnormally large caliber or volume
- abdominal pain
- bloating
- food cravings or addictions
- food aversions
- allergic shiners
- chronic sinus drainage
- red ears
- foul-smelling breath
- eczema, dry skin, or chronic rashes
- hives
- recurrent infections

- erratic behavior that may be associated with pain
- hyperactivity that may be associated with pain
- moodiness or irritability that may be associated with pain
- sleep problems that may be associated with pain

You'll want to have a record of what your child's unique signs and symptoms are at the outset of your journey toward recovery, because as you progress through the first months of your child's new GFCF diet, these are the same signs and symptoms from which your child should begin to find relief.

THE GFCF DIET

Let's start with the basics. What is gluten? What is casein? What are these two substances we are going to eliminate from your child's diet?

Gluten is a protein that is found in wheat and other grains, including oats, rye, bulgur, barley, durum, kamut, spelt, and foods made from those grains. It is also found in food starches such as semolina, couscous, and malt, in some vinegars, and in soy sauces, as well as in other flavorings. It is, for lack of more elegant words, the "sticky stuff" that binds dough together when you cook with gluten-containing flours and why, for your child's gluten-free foods made with rice or millet flours, such as your breads, pancakes, and waffle mixes, you'll be adding small amounts of binding agents such as xanthan gum.

Casein is also a protein, found in milk and foods that contain milk, such as cheese, butter, yogurt, ice cream, cottage cheese, and most brands of margarine. Casein is also often added to nonmilk products such as soy cheeses or even hot dogs in the form of *caseinate;* as you start your child on the GFCF diet, you'll learn to become an even more astute reader of food product labels to weed out key words that indicate ingredients harmful to your child.

Frequently, the names of these ingredients can be confusing—*lactides,* for example, are not dairy and are safe for our children, but *lactose* is a dairy product and may not be safe, depending on the preparation process. My amazing office manager Laurie Thomas, who has an autistic child of her own, has made grocery shopping a little easier for my patients. She has, from lists assembled by one of our families, created a set of two laminated three-by-four-inch color-coded cards (green for "go" or safe foods, and orange for "alert" or unsafe foods) that can be clipped to a key chain and taken to the supermarket for easy reference. At their first visit to my office, each parent gets a set of these cards. In the Resources section of this book, you'll find a page where these cards are reproduced; tear it out to make your own set.

All right. Now we know that GI issues are at the core of the multi-system illness we call autism. We know that restoring gut integrity is the first step in recovery—that a healthy digestive system is the proper foundation upon which to build. Why do we focus on gluten and casein? Why are they such bad things for our kids to eat? Well, because we also know that autistic children have difficulty breaking down gluten- and casein-generated *peptides*.

A peptide is a short chain of amino acids linked together. Amino acids are the main protein building blocks absorbed into the bloodstream from the gut. If only two amino acids are linked, it is called a dipeptide, and three linked amino acids is called a tripeptide, and so forth, all the way up to large polypeptide chains of around ten amino acids. The important thing to remember is that peptides, whatever their size, are also essentially proteins. Protein molecules can be digested by a human body because of the catalytic action of enzymes, which are themselves proteins. The enzymes break down the peptide chains into ever smaller lengths, with the breaks occurring at the peptide, or amino acid, bond.

Peptides either control or trigger a wide variety of functions in the human body. They act as neurotransmitters and as scavengers for free radicals; they help the bones to absorb calcium; and they flush toxins from the gall bladder, just to give you a very small idea of how vital they are to sustaining life. Glutathione, one of the most significant tools in the autism-fighting toolbox, is a critically necessary peptide. But with some peptides, as with that refreshing mug of cold beer or that tasty dish of fudge ripple ice cream, more is not always better.

Dr. Alan Friedman, a physical chemist at Johnson & Johnson, isolated and identified the peptides in the urine samples of typical and autistic children and compared the results. What he found was that the amount and volume of particles of gluten- and casein-derived peptides in the urine of autistic children were an "order of magnitude" higher than in the urine of typical children. An "order of magnitude" refers to the fixed ratio of one class of an amount to the class directly preceding it, commonly to the power of ten. What this means in the case of Dr. Friedman's study is that the autistic kids had ten times as many gluten- and casein-derived peptides as the typical kids. They were awash in peptides such as casomorphin, which can be broken down by only one known enzyme—depeptidyl peptidase IV (DPP–4)—an enzyme that we know to be either reduced or completely nonexistent in autistic kids. How damaging is a lack of DPP–4 to the human body? Well, mice who have a DPP–4 deficit will die if they are not fed a gluten-free diet. Now, performing the same experiment on human children with a similar enzyme deficiency would be terribly unethical, wouldn't it?

Autistic kids are awash in peptides such as desmorphin, which may play a role in causing the pain and spasms of the chronically elevated gut wall muscle tension many of our kids suffer and also interfere with digestion by suppressing the stimulation of gastric secretions. As in the case of casomorphin, studies are ongoing to determine the consequences of an excess of these peptides in the human system, though determining the ill effects of an overabundance of desmorphin may be a hard nut to crack as it is found in only two places in the world: on the backs of noncaptive poison dart frogs and in the urine of autistic kids.

Clearly, one of the goals of the GFCF diet is to cleanse the child's bloodstream of these harmful peptides by halting their production by the child's body.

LEAKY GUT SYNDROME

Here's your next question, I just know it: In ideal biological circumstances, these potentially harmful peptides wouldn't even stand a chance of getting into the child's bloodstream, would they?

No. And that's because the lining of the intestine is designed as a natural barrier that allows only properly digested fats and starches, as well as proteins, to pass through. Our kids, of course, don't enjoy many ideal biological circumstances. *Leaky gut syndrome,* also known more scientifically as increased intestinal permeability, is yet another of the physical problems that frequently accompany a diagnosis of autism and further complicate treatment.

Properly digested food passes through the intestine and into the bloodstream in three different ways. The first two—via "diffusion" and "active transport" through intestinal cells—concern us less in the context of autism than the third path: through *desmosomes.* Desmosomes are the spaces between the cells of the intestinal lining, and they are normally sealed tight as a drum. But when the intestinal lining is compromised through chronic inflammation, those seals loosen. Then, larger or improperly digested molecules can pass through the wall and into the blood.

But the problem doesn't stop there. These larger molecules are recognized by the body as foreign, and the immune system goes on alert to attack and kill and rid the body of what it perceives as invading giant particles. This immune defense starts yet another one of those snake-eating-its-tail cycles we talked about earlier: the longer the immune system is in attack mode, the greater is the damage done to the intestine, creating ever-larger holes in the intestinal wall; so, eventually, it is not only the bad peptides, but also larger undigested food particles and toxins that pass directly through the damaged cells and into the bloodstream. In turn, these newer, larger invaders once again trigger a now very alarmed immune system to release its heavy artillery. This escalating battle can irritate and inflame the entire body.

What makes the desmosomes loosen in the first place? What causes leaky gut syndrome? Chronic stress, intestinal infections and inflammations, POPs, bacterial overgrowth, and *poor diet*. In addition to cleansing your child's system of the unwanted peptides, the goal of the GFCF diet is to improve the nutritional quality of your child's diet so that his leaky gut can heal.

I know that the last several sections have been rather technical, filled with talk of obscure peptides and even more obscure desmosomes, minuscule components of the human body most people happily get through their whole lives without ever knowing much about. But now that you're familiar with the medical terms associated with some of the fundamental biochemical processes that go awry in our autistic kids, let's conceptualize in a much more everyday way how the GFCF diet helps to heal.

If your family is anything like mine, you prepare food for 18 to 21 meals a week in your kitchen—breakfasts, school lunches, family dinners. If you are the one who cooks these meals, you are a chemist. All food is made up of chemicals. The bright-green broccoli in your crisper, the tangy salsa and the corn chips you're going to dip in it, the nice fat chicken you just brought home from the butcher's—all technically chemicals. Through chilling, roasting, baking, or steaming, you manipulate the molecular structure of the foods to make them tastier and more nutritious, improve their texture and appearance and aroma, or preserve their freshness.

When you cook, you rely on certain conventions as you put together your family's meal. You know that when you soak black beans for chili, it not only helps to soften them and make them more digestible, but it also reduces the gas you can expect from ingesting this magical, musical legume. You know that when you sauté an onion, it gets brown and tastes sweeter because what is going on in the frying pan is the caramelization of the onion's natural sugars. You know that when you add flour to the pan drippings after you roast your chicken, the drippings get thick and you get gravy. These are all examples of the practical chemistry most of us practice at some point every day.

The biochemistry of the GFCF diet isn't as easy to see as the gravy getting thick. It takes place not in your frying pan or on your plate but at a microscopic, molecular level. But the same sorts of profoundly reliable reactions are taking place in both instances. If you squirt lemon juice on a sliced apple, the chemical reaction of the lemon juice on the apple's flesh will keep it from getting brown. But if you squirt lemon juice into a glass of milk, the milk will curdle. If you feed a child who can't tolerate casein a fresh glass of milk with dinner, her biochemistry will rebel as surely as if you'd topped off that nice cold glass of milk with a squirt of lemon juice.

THE THREE Rs

I'm going to quote my good friend the nurse Maureen McDonnell again in laying out the simplicity of the concept of the GFCF diet. In teaching parents and clinicians alike how to implement the diet, she refers to the "Three Rs"—Remove, Replenish, and Repair & Restore.

Remove the troublemaking food from the menu, especially those containing gluten and casein. I encourage my patients to begin by removing dairy and, then, within a week, to start removing food containing gluten, such as wheat flour or products made with wheat flour. I suggest using rice, potatoes, corn, and other starchy foods to make the transaction a bit easier, but keep in mind that the food sensitivities of autistic children can be fairly extensive and often extend beyond gluten and casein. It's possible, as you progress in the diet and become more and more attuned to the subtle ways your child reacts to eating certain foods, you'll want to reduce or remove these items as well.

Now, let's talk about some of the things you can expect to happen when you adhere to this new diet. You'll recall that at the beginning of Visit #1, Part 1, I mentioned that when our family began the diet with my daughter, Dani, the symptoms of her withdrawal from gluten and casein were so severe she was expelled from her school. Did you think that was odd when you read it, or perhaps an extreme reaction to having ice cream forbidden as an after-school snack and wheat sandwich bread removed from her lunch box? On the contrary, withdrawal symptoms are common when a child begins this diet, and the reason why is easy to understand. Remember the medical names for the peptides that are created in your child's body by gluten and casein? Casomorphin. Desmorphin. *Morphine.* I have seen parents balk at removing, for example, milk, from a child's diet. "Milk is good for her, isn't it? That's what we've always been told," they'll ask, but the question is often more of a demand. Then they'll add, "Besides, she *loves* milk. She drinks three or four or more glasses a day and always wants more."

Exactly.

She craves it. Those peptides are creating an opiate-like reaction in her body. It is fairly typical to see symptoms similar to opiate withdrawal, and to even see regression, during the first few days of the diet, as your child overcomes her addiction. Hang in there. It usually lasts for only a few days. It gets better.

Replenish the probiotics—the good gut bacteria that facilitate digestion but whose numbers may have been severely diminished in the child's system through overuse of the antibiotics (and the development of dysbiosis) children receive so frequently to treat infections. Good sources of probiotics are cultured vegetables, nondairy yogurt, and young coconut kefir. But a good clinician will make giving probiotics a bit easier on a family that is guiding a child in a whole new way of eating and may find the child not only resistant to new foods—as children everywhere can be to some degree—but also battling with withdrawal symptoms. I recommend a daily dose or doses of bottled probiotics for my patients. The warning here is that some probiotics contain dairy, so be sure to check the ingredient label to make sure your brand is nondairy.

Replenish enzymes lining the gut wall microscopically and frequently absent in the inflamed organs we see on endoscopies. Initially, we use enzymes added to meals and snacks, much as we do with children who have cystic fibrosis. And sometimes, we even use the same enzymes those children do. But, more often, we choose enzymes specially designed for children who are not making the DPP–4 that can break up the morphine-like peptides that are so troublesome to them. As the gut heals, and the gut lining can once again make its own enzymes, there may be less need for added enzymes over time.

Replenish the vitamins, minerals, and omega fatty acids that may be missing from your child's diet or that have not been adequately absorbed by a diseased bowel. Your clinician may not go into this phase of replenishment with you in much depth until your second consultation. This is standard practice for me. By the second visit, I have laboratory results that allow me to pinpoint much more accurately which essential elements are missing from the child's chemistry and need to be supplemented. I do recommend, however, that every child start out by supplementing these basics as long as they are well tolerated:

- a good multivitamin that is rich in B complex
- omega fatty acids, usually cod liver oil made by a company that removes the organs before they press the flesh of the fish (this minimizes toxicities from the fish itself)
- probiotics
- vitamin D_3, starting at just 1,000 IU daily until we have levels measured
- digestive enzymes containing DPP–4 with each meal
- melatonin, if sleep is a big issue.

Repair & restore the myriad of building blocks that our children cannot or do not ingest, absorb, or utilize effectively. Please note that the supplements I've listed above are the basics; you can find more information about these basics, as well as the range of tools in the supplement toolbox, beginning on page 102.

By starting your child on the GFCF diet; supplementing essential vitamins, minerals, and fatty acids; and adding probiotics and enzymes, you have started on your way toward normalizing the usually subtle, but quite significant, abnormalities in his biochemical system that have resulted in the diagnosis of autism. You have begun the healing.

VISIT #1

ACTION LIST

Start your child—and maybe even your whole family—on the GFCF diet.

While it may be unrealistic to expect your entire family to take this novel dietary path, the benefits of introducing everyone to more whole foods should be obvious. In my case, we began the GFCF diet as a family unit out of, I suppose, solidarity with Dani, so that she wouldn't feel singled out or deprived.

What we quickly came to realize is that the GFCF diet is not about deprivation. Focus not on what is gone, but on what is left. The foods are really quite delicious, and there really is a great variety of food that is diet-legal once you grow comfortable with exploring all the options available. Visit some (or all) of the websites listed in the Resources section of this book for helpful tips on GFCF-approved ingredients, cooking tips, and recipes.

Search out alternatives for foods your family really likes.

In our house the problem was Cheetos. The kids loved them. It might have been torture for Dani to sit with her brother and watch a football game while he munched on the snack food that she was forbidden. Fortunately, there is a product called Tings, a Cheetos-like snack with none of the gluten or casein—none of the junk—but all of the taste. Both of my kids have actually come to prefer them.

Join a GFCF support group.

There are many to be found locally these days, and the Talk About Curing Autism (TACA) chapters springing up nationwide are supportive of dietary and medical intervention. Visit them at www.talkaboutcuringautism.org to see if there's a chapter near you. The diet, especially as you make your initial transition into a new way of cooking and eating, can seem like a lot of work. Networking with parents who have been there and done that can relieve a lot of the stress associated with the lifestyle change you are making for your child. Experienced parents can talk you through the hard parts and the down times and help you remember, through relating their own experience, that better days are on their way.

Keep a diary.

Go out to your local office supply store and buy a composition book or a steno pad, or to your stationery store for a fancier blank book, or start a new spreadsheet on your computer if you prefer to keep your diary electronically. The crucial thing is that you keep an ongoing record of your child's progress through the biomedical intervention. *Write things down.* Relying on your recollections is an iffy proposition, especially regarding something as emotionally charged as your child's health.

Record what your child is eating, what supplements she is taking, and how he is reacting to each new addition or subtraction from his regimen. It is important to remember that each autistic child will recover differently, because each child's biochemistry is uniquely impacted. Your child may, after a few days of withdrawal, suddenly start sleeping through the night, and you may attribute this blessing to the removal of casein and gluten from the table. But then, one day, she may suddenly experience a recurrence of the insomnia. You'll look in your diary and discover that this was the day you began B complex vitamins. In this case, you'll want to reduce the dosage, or perhaps stop the B complex altogether, but you will want to feel confident that it was the B complex vitamin that caused the problem. This is an example of the sort of detailed observation that will help you and your clinician find the right balance of foods and supplements for your child's one-of-a-kind biochemistry. By referring to your records, you can more easily tie together action and consequence.

The entries you make in the diary don't have to be elaborate. "Started Johnny today on one tablespoon of probiotics in the morning and one at night." "Sarah 'accidentally' ate a wheat cookie. Her teacher told me the class was celebrating someone's birthday, and she didn't think one cookie would hurt. Had a talk with her to explain that, yes, it did hurt and why. I don't think there will be any more 'accidents.' This morning took a box of GFCF cookies for the teacher to keep in her desk for such occasions, just to make sure." "Today, Eric refused to take his DMG [dimethylglycine], and by this evening, the whole family could tell he was out of sorts. We were all stepping around like we were on eggshells again. Am going to hide the DMG in his juice tomorrow and see if that works." You can go into more detail if you'd like, but these sorts of short notations are just fine too. Your diary is going to be one of the most useful resources you and your clinician will have in achieving the subtle balance of foods, supplements, and other therapies that will heal your child.

Record your child's behaviors in the diary as well, the indicators of improvement you will see in your child as you progress on the diet. You'll likely be pleased to note

- improvement in bowel function and stool consistency;
- a decrease in crying and screaming, which are usually indicators of pain, so you'll be able to tell whether the diet is soothing your child's suffering;
- improvement in emotional regulation;
- improvement in cognition.

I'll stress again that the diary you are going to keep is going to be an important reference for you and your doctor as you move through the biomedical protocol. It will eliminate any guesswork in deciding what is the best course for your child's treatment—and it will be a permanent document of your child's joyful gains in overall health and happiness.

Try to buy organic and local foods, as the family food budget will allow.

Remember this as you shop: there is often a huge difference between the *cost* of something and its *value*. For the sake of keeping the numbers simple, say that the cost of a can of spinach to feed your family is $2, while the cost of an equivalent amount of fresh spinach from your local organic greengrocer is $3. The organic spinach, which, as we discussed earlier, provides up to twice the content of vitamins and minerals as the canned vegetable, has value that more than makes up for the difference in cost.

Use up your old, chemical-based cleaning fluids and replace them with organic cleaning agents.

If—heaven forbid—someone in your household still smokes cigarettes, cigars, or pipes, I'm going to assume that, like most everyone else today, you've mandated that as an exclusively outdoor activity.

In any case, though actually stopping as you're getting through starting a new diet may not be the right time, now is definitely the time to renew your commitment to quit. I nag any of my patients' smoking parents gently but continually until they quit. When they do, we do the Snoopy Happy Dance in the office.

Be strict about the diet.

I couldn't possibly stress this point enough, so I'm just going to repeat it: be strict about the diet. There isn't room here for "just one cookie" or "just one scoop of ice cream." One cookie or one scoop will do harm. Think of it this way: when an alcoholic decides to become sober, no one in his right mind would tell him that just one sip of wine won't matter. That's because we all know that to an alcoholic, the wine or beer or whiskey he prefers is poison, given his unique biochemistry. In the process of detoxifying his system from alcohol, the alcoholic's biochemistry is slowly rebalancing itself; giving in to one craving for a drink throws the balance once again into chaos. Remember also that casein and gluten are relatively pro-inflammatory molecules that perpetuate that chronic inflammatory process we're trying to mitigate. Even if there aren't huge negative behaviors associated with feeding your child these foods, they may still be generating inflammation in the bowel and body of your child.

Don't throw your child's biochemical balance back into chaos. Don't perpetuate the inflammation. Stock up on the very tasty GFCF brand cookies and ice creams. Ask to be notified about any parties at her school—the sort of parties where cupcakes are typically served—and plan ahead; send a GFCF cupcake to school that day with your child so that she can participate in the celebration too without compromising her health. Talk to your child's teachers, and to his friends' parents; enlist their support in helping your child maintain the diet that is critical to his recovery.

Make a videotape of your child before starting the diet and supplements.

I have had patients finally get to the diagnostic doctor's visit long after starting the diet, and their dramatically improved child no longer meets the criteria for ASD. A videotape helps those physicians to see the disease in its untreated form without having to experience it again at home and at school. It also helps family members to stay the dietary course, to stay on the dietary wagon, when their memories of the nightmare behaviors fade and they are ready to give back the gluten and casein.

Cultivate patience.

Sometimes the rewards of the GFCF diet will be huge and readily apparent—a teacher will go out of his way to telephone you because he must remark on your son's dramatic improvement in concentration in the classroom, or your daughter, who has been indifferent to human contact for months, will quietly snuggle up next to you for a hug while you're watching TV. For those of us who are parents of autistic kids, these are events worthy of fireworks and parades and brass bands.

But there are smaller rewards too—that first day with a normal poop, or the sudden realization upon looking in your food diary that it's been a month since he's had any sort of sinus issue. Look for these small rewards along the way and allow yourself and your child the opportunity to savor them. Pace yourself, because recovery from autism is not a sprint, it's a marathon. Taking the full measure of joy from every milestone achievement, small or large, refreshes you and your child and keeps you energized for the long haul.

"MOMMY, I HAVE FLEAS"

YEAST, LABS, AND SUPPLEMENTS

JUSTIN

Ordinarily, I try to see my patients about every two months at first. As they improve, I see them less frequently. Those of us with autistic kids in our lives know, however, that our lives are rarely anything like ordinary, so the two-month time period between visits, while providing a framework within which to plan, is merely an estimate. I ask my patients' parents to schedule their return visits on a case-by-case basis, depending on the severity of the individual child's illness and how I can project his progress through the treatment approach.

Ideally, enough time has elapsed between visits so that the child, the parents, and I will be able not only to see some gains being made because of adherence to the GFCF diet, but also to pinpoint which parts of the treatment are working best for this inimitable child. Through the record you have kept in your treatment journal, we will be able to track the child's responses to the removal of casein. Then we can gauge any new reactions once the gluten has been removed and, specifically, to each addition and sometimes dosage change of different vitamins, minerals, enzymes, and probiotics.

I have to tell you that more often than not, there are reasons to take pleasure out of these subsequent meetings with my patients and their parents. The parents come into my office with smiles on their faces and pull out their diaries, notebooks, or computer printouts, eager to tell me about the ways in which their child has regained some of her health and skills since we've last met. I never cut short this time of sharing joy—it's a time of affirmation that nourishes the whole treatment team.

But I also have to tell you that as I rejoice with the parents, I keep a close eye on the child, who is usually out in my waiting room playing with the stuffed animals or with the train village. Often, what I note when I observe the kids coming back for their second visit is undeniable evidence of the next hurdle we have to clear on our long marathon: yeast.

Yeast is a little microbe that makes us itch. Those little critters that are not considered normal anywhere in the body when they begin to multiply in significant numbers. When Dani got enough language back to start to tell me what was wrong, she often told me: "I have fleas." I chronicled her progress by the way she communicated this to me over the first many months: "Mommy, I have fleas again." "Mommy, I have fleas, please call Dr. Jerry." "Mommy, I have fleas, did you ask Dr. Jerry for Diflucan?" and finally, "Mommy, PUHLEEZ call Dr. Jerry, I have GOT to have Diflucan for these FLEAS!" Thankfully, yeast is controlled much better these days; she knows so much about how to manage it that she can just about call the pharmacy directly.

When Justin walked into my office for his second visit, almost two months had gone by since I'd last seen him. He'd celebrated his fourth birthday since his last appointment. His parents were thrilled with his progress on the GFCF diet. In many ways, this was indeed a different child I was seeing.

Justin was much more verbal, for one thing, able to converse with me, albeit in quick, blunt exchanges. His excrement, though still fairly watery and unformed and stinky, was no longer explosive, and his bowel movements were coming at predictable intervals. He was coming along so well with potty training, in fact, that his parents were hopeful he'd soon graduate from diapers. He had started out fiercely resisting his twice-daily doses of supplements but, over the course of several weeks, had settled down and now took them more or less willingly. This was a change that we might have attributed to simple resignation—his parents were adamant that he was going to take the supplements, and he himself had grown weary of fighting them about it—but his mom had a different theory. She'd noticed that on the days when the daily fights had ended with Justin successfully ingesting the supplements, his screaming and tantrum throwing were significantly curtailed. She speculated that this was because the supplements were doing their biochemical work effectively and Justin just felt better. He was less uncomfortable and, so, less irritable, and—here is her crucial point—Justin *himself* had noticed it. He hadn't come to like taking the supplements, but he had made the connection between taking them and feeling better.

Justin's mom told me this almost shyly, worried that in her own enthusiasm she was reading too much into Justin's change of heart, but hers is a position with which I tend to agree. Time after time, I have seen autistic kids grow not only to accept but also to look forward to taking their supplements, as well as undergoing other treatments. These kids, as I've pointed out before, are rarely mentally deficient no matter how blank their facial expressions may appear; they hear every word I say about making their tummies feel better, about making their heads stop hurting. The lively, curious minds beneath the fog are perfectly capable of making what is, after all, a relatively basic association: if I do "a" then "b" will occur; when I receive treatment for my illness, I feel better.

YEAST

The area where Justin had made no significant progress was in controlling his hyperactivity, or his spinning. He was still a veritable whirligig, climbing everywhere and waking up at night laughing hysterically, his parents told me, spinning and spinning in circles, and they had no difficulty in proving it: Justin was in my waiting room giggling up a storm while trying to whirl a hole through the floor. It was easy to recognize what I have come to know as the classic symptoms of chronic yeast.

In our guts, most of us humans have some yeast—commonly a yeast form known as candida. Whether or not this truly is "normal," I'm not sure, but it certainly is accepted as the norm these days. The yeast is kept under control in a healthy gut, with a healthy immune system, by naturally occurring probiotics such as lactobacillus and bifidobacteria. Yeast not well controlled grows exponentially. Provided the correct environment, it may ferment the sugars it is fed in your child's gut, much like a barrel of wine or a keg of beer. That notorious gut-brain connection can then make our children seem drunk, or foggy. When yeast dies, it releases myriad toxins that biochemically make us feel lousy, or itchy, or rashy—as if we might have fleas.

Like so many autistic kids, Justin had suffered from recurring infections—in his case, recurring earaches—and had almost constantly in his young life been on one course of antibiotics or another. Antibiotics, as I've already said, can be life savers. Certainly, they kill off infection. But at the same time as they kill off the bacteria that made us ill, they also kill off the good bacteria in our systems. One of the things the good bacteria do is contain yeast so that it doesn't become excessive. When the number of good bacteria is diminished, yeast begins to thrive.

What else can allow yeast overgrowth? An environment that selects yeast—that preferentially allows yeast to grow—is one that is highly sugared, more acidic, has less oxygen, and is immunologically less competent. This environment prevents bacteria from growing as well, leaving more room for the yeast.

It is not surprising, in this age of antibiotics, that most of us, children and adults alike, will experience some form of yeast infection—especially if we don't accompany a course of antibiotics with extra intake of probiotics of the sort found in nondairy yogurt. Have you ever had a vaginal yeast infection? Athlete's foot? "Jock itch"? A discolored yellow toenail? These are all indicative of infestations of excessive yeast in the body. The intensity of these common infestations can cause symptoms that range from a mild but constant itch on the surface of the skin or affected tissue, to a deeper itch that feels as if it is under the skin or inside the tissue, to dangerous infection and inflammation.

In a child with autism, whose need for and use of antibiotics has historically been well above the average, or whose immune system has become dysfunctional, the yeast can grow out of control and take up permanent residence in his system. When the yeast—and it's important to note that our children often harbor other strains of fungi besides just candida—has been around long enough, it turns into a particularly aggressive fungal form, *mycelia*. Mycelia molecules are barbed, toxic, and ridiculously hard to kill. To the child infested to this stage with yeast, the itching he experiences is continuous and can be almost too much to bear, a constant crawling sensation under his skin and within his muscles.

There are many symptoms a trained clinician will look for in determining if the child is experiencing a systemic overgrowth of yeast, though some of them, like Justin's hyperactivity, spinning, and inappropriate laughter, are readily apparent to clinician and non-clinician alike. Other symptoms to look for are

- skin rashes
- thrush, or a thick white coating in the mouth, particularly the tongue
- insomnia and other sleep problems
- abdominal pain
- digestive distress, including bloating, gas, and diarrhea
- swelling, particularly in the face, hands, and/or feet
- chronic water retention

- otherwise unexplained fatigue or depression
- nasal congestion or swelling of the nasal membranes
- a history of steroid or antibiotic use
- muscle aches
- joint pain
- headaches
- weight gain
- cravings for sweets or other carbohydrates.

The symptoms of systemic yeast overgrowth, furthermore, include some of those signs and symptoms that are often conventionally used to confirm a diagnosis of true autism:

- poor memory
- poor cognitive function
- brain or mental fog
- extreme sensitivity—to sound (of the sort that causes the child to cower and cover her ears with her hands), to hair and nail cutting, or to teeth brushing
- self-injurious behavior such as head banging and scratching.

Indeed, Justin was scratching at his belly in between spinning his circles, and when I asked him if he would show me where he was itchy, he pulled up his shirt and I saw the bloody streaks his fingernails had made in his flesh in a desperate attempt to relieve the terrible crawling sensation.

These types of deep, self-inflicted scratches are not uncommon in autistic kids. But they are *not* mindless attempts to hurt themselves. They are the result of trying to find relief. Restlessness, anger, extreme agitation, hair-trigger tempers, and aggression are also often listed as symptoms of a systemic yeast infection, but, more realistically, these behaviors come about simply because most autistic children don't have the verbal skills to tell you that it feels as if an army of very active little insects has lodged itself deep inside their bodies, and the insects are having one hell of a wild party in there. The child will, instead, continue to try to just scratch away the pain and discomfort, and the results are the alarming-looking wounds he creates on his skin.

YEAST DAMAGE

Why does the scratching that frequently accompanies a systemic yeast infection look so gruesome? Well, in part, because the itch is deep, and so it feels to the sufferer that the accompanying scratch must be deep as well in order to offer any sort of satisfaction. In greater part, it is because the yeast-infected skin is just not as structurally sound as normal skin.

When you scratch a patch of normal, healthy skin, the abrasive action relieves the temporary agitation of the cell or cells that got a little jumpy. But yeast that has been in residence in living tissue for a while will actually send out "roots" and start to bore into the tissue. This compromises the structure of the tissue, so even mild scratching can result in breaking the skin and in bleeding.

These yeast "roots" do not cause problems only on the surface of the skin, however. They spread into whatever tissue they happen to live in—commonly, mucus membranes that are found in the mouth and genital areas and in the intestinal walls—compromising the integrity of those tissues as well. These areas, too, can become inflamed and infected as the yeast roots, slowly but insidiously, settle into the host tissue for the long haul. As the roots spread and settle, they start to displace the tissue's healthy cells, even poking holes in the membrane to gain and strengthen their foothold in the tissue.

Holes in the intestinal walls? Yes. And that means just what you suspect it does: the yeast infestation can become a contributing cause of the leaky gut syndrome we've already talked about, or it can exacerbate the permeability of an already-unhealthy gut and worsen the existing leaky gut syndrome caused by the child's other malfunctioning biochemical reactions. This worsening allows even more partially or completely undigested proteins to leak into the child's bloodstream, triggers the dysfunctional immune system to an even higher level of dysfunctional activity, and causes the production of neurotoxins that lead to even more of the erratic behaviors and cognitive dysfunctions we recognize as autism. As you can see, yeast infestations can set off another of the snake-eating-its-tail cycles that have to be broken for the child to heal.

It was not only Justin's tummy that was scratched up. I lifted his shirt up a bit further and saw that his armpits were nearly shredded. The areas of his body where the yeast was causing him the most intense problems were important, as was the time of the year of his visit to me—August, a month that is hot and humid where we live in Florida. One tell-tale sign of yeast is that it likes a hot, humid, friendly environment. Depending on the season of the year and the climate in which you live, yeast infections can seem like an epidemic when one is working with autistic kids.

"Okay, Justin," I said to this little guy, holding his hands in a friendly but firm grasp to try to prevent him from tearing into this armpits once again, "we're going to make it so it doesn't itch you anymore, all right?"

Justin was trying to wiggle his hands free of mine, but he was also looking straight at me with perfect understanding, and hope.

TREATING YEAST

There are many reasons we struggle so much with yeast in my practice. The yeast has had a significant head start on my efforts to quell it. There are many strains that are only sensitive to one antifungal. The environment that is so inviting to them heals slowly, and until the gut is in better shape, yeast overgrowth will continue to be favored. That's why I recommend being very aggressive with any yeast infection.

The place to begin treating yeast is with the child's diet. Let's go right to your pantry to make the reason why crystal clear. You get up in the morning to brew your first cup of coffee. You open the cupboard where you keep your coffee-making equipment—your tin of ground coffee, your filters, and your sugar bowl—and you are greeted by the unwelcome sight of a line of ants marching to and from that sugar bowl. Someone left the lid off the bowl overnight, and these enterprising insects have found a delightful new food source. What's the first thing you do? Right, remove the sugar bowl—remove the ant's food source.

Sugar is also a food source for yeast. In order to kill the yeast that is invading the child's body, we need to eliminate what is feeding it and keeping it alive. The less sugar and the fewer high-glycemic carbohydrates (those that turn most easily into sugar)—especially potatoes and rice—the child eats, the less there is for the yeast to eat too.

There are many books that have been written exclusively about the yeast-fighting diet, and there are many websites that can concisely guide you through the diet as well. Rather than adhere rigidly to a second diet, I try to incorporate some of the approach into our GFCF diet. Let me just lay out a few of the fundamentals here.

Sugar needs to be drastically reduced in most children's diets, and that means sugar in all its forms: simple sugars—sucrose, fructose, lactose, maltose, glucose, mannitol, and sorbital—and other sugar products such as maple syrup and molasses. Look, as well, for any of the sugars to be avoided on the ingredient labels of any packaged or processed foods. Although you will have eliminated a lot of packaged foods from your child's diet already, because you are already adhering to the GFCF diet and incorporating more and more whole and organic foods into your meals, you will still be surprised at how many products contain some form of added sugar. It's not only the breakfast cereals aimed at the youth market and sweet snack foods you need to watch out for, as "yeast friendly" is a term that could easily be substituted for "kid friendly." Baked beans, most condiments, pickles, hot dogs, and bacon are just a few of the products that can contain sugar of one sort or another. When you need to use a little sugar for something, try to make it one that isn't processed, and is natural—like honey, agave nectar, and rapidura or other more raw sugars. Fruits can be used as well, but the tendency to overuse fruit when children would like to avoid veggies is very tempting. Stevia and Xylitol are also acceptable sweeteners, and Xylitol appears to have the added benefit of helping to keep our teeth healthier.

You'll want to avoid food and drinks that concentrate natural sugars, such as packaged fruit juices and most dried fruits. If you think that you yourself have some of the symptoms of a yeast overgrowth and you want to cleanse your own system as well, remember that alcoholic drinks—beer, wine, cider, and other, harder alcoholic beverages—contain sugar and will need to be eliminated. Now it is worth noting, as a parent, after surviving a long day of getting your autistic, only-white-food-crosses-my-lips child onto a GFCF, low-sugar, healthy, as-organic-as-possible diet, that a glass of wine can be very therapeutic—I like a glass of wine once in a while myself. But if you are experiencing a yeast infestation, wine, too, alas, has sugar, and needs to go. I know these dietary changes are hard. We did it in my house. We still do it at my house. And it is worth doing.

Foods you'll want to be moderate about consuming include even the grains that are legal on the GFCF diet and certain high-carbohydrate vegetables such as sweet corn, potatoes, even peas and beans. Fresh fruit juices should also be restricted because of their high sugar content. Remember that we were designed to consume water. The only fruit juice there was before the Industrial Revolution was manually squeezed.

YEAST-FIGHTING AGENTS

I am a proponent of herbal and homeopathic methods for fighting yeast. Herbal concoctions were the original pharmaceuticals, after all, and we can still turn to a lot of these natural remedies with a great deal of confidence. In fact, where there is a choice between a natural herbal formula that is well tolerated and effective and a chemical pharmaceutical, I am going to be among the first to recommend sticking with the natural herbal product. The list of antifungal herbals is extensive—barberry, olive leaf extract, garlic, goldenseal, Oregon grape root, oregano oil, peppermint oil, and rosemary, to name but a few. There are several good antiyeast capsules and teas on the market that combine these and other ingredients into effective medicine. In addition, I will often recommend a daily dose of aloe vera juice, which not only assists the body in killing off yeast, but also helps to move constipated bowels.

I am also open to discussing the use of homeopathic treatments for yeast in relation to how these alternative remedies can complement, without compromising, the total biomedical intervention process—and a credible homeopathic practitioner is going to insist you consult with a medical doctor for advice on managing any concurrent illnesses anyway.

Homeopathy may seem counterintuitive to some people as it uses "like to cure like." That is, if you or your child is suffering from a candida yeast infestation, the homeopath will use a miniscule dose of candida in the remedy. If the patient—or, in my case, the patient's parents—find their comfort level within the "like to cure like" philosophy, and if the recommended treatment will not interfere with the progress of the biomedical protocol, then homeopathy can be a good optional extra in the goal of killing yeast. One thing I do warn my patients about, however, when they decide on homeopathy, is that they need to be cautious about buying homeopathic remedies over the Internet. One reason for this is that the practice of homeopathy is a fairly complex skill that considers the mental and emotional health of the patient in prescribing custom-designed remedies. If you are interested in pursuing this course of treatment as an additional yeast-fighting tool, you are better off finding a homeopathic practitioner or naturopath who will personally guide the treatment and is willing to work in tandem with your regular practitioner.

All of that said—all of my personal confidence in the efficacy of some herbal and homeopathic treatments for some patients on the record—I want to make it clear that when the situation warrants it, I am pretty quick to prescribe antifungal pharmaceuticals. If the yeast is out of control in the child's body, our best course of action is to get it under control with as little delay as possible. Pharmaceuticals are often simply the most rapid and most effective choice. The bottom line is that the more quickly we can decrease the yeast, the more quickly the child will find relief from that incessant itch that is tormenting him and the more quickly those symptoms of autism that are associated with a yeast overgrowth—such as short tempers that lead to tantrums, poor cognition, and mental fog—will begin to decrease as well.

For this reason, I will often advise parents who want to go the herbal or homeopathic route to begin their child on a course of antifungal drugs and, as the yeast is reduced, start the alternative treatments, eventually weaning the child from the drugs and onto the strictly herbal and/or homeopathic path.

By your second visit with your biomedical practitioner, the lab results from the blood, urine, and stool samples you collected the first time around will be back and sitting in front of the doctor. The results will often provide the concrete evidence of yeast infection and help to direct selection of an appropriate pharmaceutical antifungal.

YEAST DIE-OFF

Yeast "die-off" is the general, popular term used to describe what some medical doctors will refer to as *Herxheimer reaction*. Die-off simply describes what happens when pathogenic organisms die en masse in the body; unfortunately, dealing with the body's reaction to the mass death is not so simple.

When yeast dies off in the body, a host of symptoms may manifest, the most discouraging of which is that the symptoms of yeast infestation that the patient is already experiencing may spike sharply. You see, the symptoms of a yeast infestation are caused in the first place by the living, yeast-releasing by-products of its metabolism, and these by-products are toxic. When you kill the yeast, the microbes will release even greater amounts of those toxins. It takes time for the dead yeast cells, as well as the toxins they create, to be eliminated from the body, and during that time, symptoms can become heightened.

I know, I know; right about now that feels like just more bad news, doesn't it? But here's the good news: the increased release of the toxins is only temporary. While it can take anywhere from four to six months to get an advanced yeast infestation well under control, and the die-off reaction can come and go during this period, the reaction lasts typically for only one day to one week.

Most everyone will, at some point or points in the yeast-killing process, experience a die-off reaction, and for most everyone the die-off will manifest in a different combination of symptoms, such as

- fatigue
- mental fog
- nausea
- bloating
- diarrhea or constipation
- excessive gas
- headaches
- sore throats
- increased itching
- increased muscle or joint pain or discomfort
- low-grade fever
- the standard, punky feeling you get when you are coming down with the flu.

Autistic kids are, unfortunately, likely to experience these symptoms even more intensely than otherwise healthy people who are cleansing yeast because the heavy metals that are already in autistic systems can cause special problems. Autistic kids can experience extra strain on the organs that are trying to eliminate the dead yeast cells and the yeast toxins from the body—the liver, the kidneys, the colon, and the lymphatic system. That is why, with autistic kids, it is especially important to kill the yeast in stages, or phases, to help assuage the discomfort they may experience, and to keep precise track in your journal of your child's reactions along the way.

Is your child experiencing a great deal of nausea, or running a low-grade fever? Then cut back on the dose of antifungal agents you are using for a few days and work it back up gradually.

Killing yeast is in no way a race to see who can best endure and overcome those symptoms I've just mentioned. On the contrary, those symptoms are *not* a sign that yeast is dying, but that the child's body is on detox overload—that his systems are working far too hard to deal with a toxic crisis and they can't cope. The symptoms of die-off are signs that you need to back off just slightly from your yeast-killing efforts and give her body the time it needs to catch up with all you are asking it to do.

There are, as well, several other things that you can do to help soothe your child's symptoms and help him to cope. Encourage him to drink a lot of filtered water—preferably warm or room temperature—because it will help flush the dead yeast cells and their toxins from his system. Allow him all the rest that he desires; killing yeast is going to tax his systems, and he will likely be fatigued at some point in the process; keep his schedule flexible to allow for naps if he needs them—unlike most kids at naptime, he will be grateful for it. Draw him lots of baths and pour a cup of Epsom salts in the water, sometimes several times daily. An occasional dose of ibuprofen (of the dye- and sugar-free sort) can soothe the discomfort, and sometimes we even use a little activated charcoal to draw the toxins from the bloodstream into the gut for excretion.

Sometimes, killing yeast will make a child constipated, and this is an especially unwanted symptom of die-off, as dead yeast cells tend to accumulate behind the retained fecal matter and in the mucous lining of the bowel. This is where some aloe juice, some fiber, or even, on occasion, a glycerin suppository can be helpful.

Through the process of yeast killing, make sure that you don't run out of any of the bottled probiotics your child may be taking. Probiotics are particularly important at this time. When the yeast dies, probiotics actually fill in the physical spaces left by the abandoned yeast colonies and, so, help to ease the die-off reaction.

YEAST AND THE IMMUNE SYSTEM

The length of time that it takes to cleanse your child's body of unwanted yeast, and the intensity and frequency of the die-off reaction she will experience while you're treating the yeast infestation, will depend largely on two main things: the degree of infestation—that is, how much yeast she is hosting and how long the yeast has been there—and the strength of her immune system.

Now, we all know that autistic kids don't enjoy generally healthy immune systems to start with. How do we help them compensate for this deficit? One of the methods I have used successfully is a course of the pharmaceutical *low-dose Naltrexone* (LDN).

Okay. I'm a doctor, and doctors are not, as a group, temperamentally given to hyperbole. I am also personally conscious of the admonition that with every blessing there can come a curse. LDN has been called by some a miracle drug. Don't believe it; those things don't exist. I'm telling you this right up front, because after I tell you a little bit about LDN, you might be tempted to think of it in those terms, and as with anything you put into your child's body—or your own body, for that matter—especially anything *chemical,* the consideration you give to it has to be very clearheaded and practical. You have to find your comfort zone with any new drug before you can confidently add it to your child's regimen. After I talk with my patient's parents about any new pharmaceutical, I urge them to do their homework—in this case to go to www.low dosenaltrexone.org to read up on the drug—before they make a decision whether or not to try it with their child. What follows in the next few paragraphs is a condensed and paraphrased version of what you'll find on the site.

Naltrexone is a drug that was approved by the Food and Drug Administration (FDA) in 1984 for the purpose of helping heroin and opium addicts. Naltrexone blocks the effects of the these drugs by blocking the user's opioid receptors. In 1985, Dr. Bernard Bihari, a physician with a clinical practice in New York City, discovered the effects of a much smaller dose of Naltrexone on the body's immune system. He found that low doses, taken at bedtime, were able to enhance a patient's response to infection by HIV, the virus that causes AIDS. In the mid-1990s, Dr. Bihari found that patients in his practice who were suffering with various cancers and autoimmune diseases such as lupus also often showed prompt control of the disease activity while taking LDN.

Up to the present time, the question "What controls the immune system?" has not been comprehensively answered in the curricula of medical colleges, and the issue has not formed a part of the received wisdom of practicing physicians. In all fairness, this is in part because our understanding of the immune system, a tremendously complex entity, is expanding exponentially. Nonetheless, a body of research over the past two decades has pointed repeatedly to one's own endorphin secretions (or internal opioids) as playing the central role in the beneficial orchestration of the immune system. The brief blocking of opioid receptors in LDN users between 2 A.M. and 4 A.M. that is caused by taking LDN at bedtime each night is believed to produce a prolonged up-regulation of vital elements of the immune system by causing an increase in endorphin and enkephalin production.

In short, as it says on the site, LDN boosts the immune system by activating the body's own natural defenses. Not only has it been used successfully as part of the treatment of addictions, HIV, various cancers, and lupus, but it has also eased the suffering of patients with Lou Gehrig's disease, Alzheimer's, celiac disease, Crohn's disease, irritable bowel syndrome, multiple sclerosis, Parkinson's, and rheumatoid arthritis, to name but a few diseases with autoimmune components. It has also, of course, been used successfully in the treatment of ASD to help regulate our kids' immune systems.

If, as a clinician, I discern that LDN may be appropriate for your child, I am apt to ask you to go home and study the website and talk with your partner about its potential benefits in your child's unique condition. If you feel LDN is right for your child, at that point I am happy to write a prescription.

If I seem overly cautious, part of the reason may be that when we have finished our discussion of yeast and treatment for it, the parents and I are likely to launch right into a detailed discussion of dietary supplements. You see, this discussion of yeast ordinarily takes place on the second visit, and by the second visit, the test results for the child's blood, urine, and stool samples are available for us to dissect minutely. We are probably going to add to the list of supplements the child should be taking and adjust the doses of even the ones she is currently taking. In order that the parents aren't overwhelmed by the sheer number of capsules, chewables, and supplement drops our approach requires them to give to their child often twice each day, it's important that they feel they are in control and understand, by education, the choices we as a team are making to restore their child's health. I believe that thorough transparency is really the only way parents can be the thoughtful, confident partners in recovery their child needs them to be.

ONE LAST WORD ABOUT YEAST, AND STRESS

Please recall what I said about the symptoms of die-off: they are *not* evidence of an efficient and fast-working cleanse; rather, they are evidence that the child's body is being overtaxed, asked to do too much all at once, and needs a rest. Go into the phase of killing yeast knowing that you'll need extra stores of patience. The treatment is commonly of the two steps forward, one step back variety, and your child may well become cranky or even show signs of real regression through the process. Take heart: both of these things are normal and to be expected. They can, however, be mitigated with the additional measures I have just discussed. But if you accept up front that there are going to be setbacks, you are less likely to become stressed about them.

Stress.

Everyday stress, as you'll recall I've already said, can be one of the contributors to oxidative stress, and oxidative stress is a condition to which everyone, not just our kids, is susceptible. Stress exacerbates and worsens almost every health concern. Everyday stress, as a matter of fact, can also contribute to a less efficient yeast detox. It benefits your child in so many ways to be surrounded by calm and confidence as much as that is at all possible during his healing time—and it is especially important that he feels this calm, confident stability from the parents who care for him daily, because *stress is contagious.* To that end, Mom and Dad, please remember that you are a much more effective partner in your child's recovery when you are yourselves rested and feeling whole—and what this sometimes means is that you have to look after yourselves first, so that your child doesn't "catch" your stress and become "infected" by it.

Think of it this way: when you are on an airplane, the flight attendants appear before takeoff and run through a short safety speech most of us have heard so many times we don't even listen to it anymore. But one of the safety procedures that is always mentioned concerns those yellow oxygen masks that are supposed to drop from above our seat in case the cabin loses air pressure. The flight attendants instruct the passengers that should those masks drop during the flight, adults should put their face masks on first before attempting to help a child who may be traveling with them.

These instructions, upon first hearing, might see counterintuitive to us. Aren't we always supposed to put our children's welfare first? Of course. But in the event you're in an airplane during an emergency depressurization situation, in order to best help your child you have to be able to breathe yourself. In this situation, you *are* putting the child's needs first by making sure you're calm, reasoned, and able to effectively assist him with his own mask.

As you run the long marathon of recovery with your child, remember to put on your own mask first—or, at least, from time to time, remember to put it on at all. This means that sometimes, the primary caregiver—usually Mom—needs a day off to go to lunch with her girlfriends, get a manicure, simply curl up and read a book, or quietly close her eyes. Somebody to spot her with child care for even a few hours can profoundly and positively influence her sense of well-being—a sense of well-being that contributes more directly than you might realize to your child's own sense of God's in his heaven and all's right with the world.

It also means that Mom and Dad need a night off together every once in a while. *Alone.* No kids. Date night. I cannot tell you how many times I have written prescriptions to the parents for a date together. I've forbidden them from coming back until they can tell me about the movie they saw on their date. Yes, it might feel awkward and worrisome the first night Mom and Dad go out without the kids. It might feel selfish to indulge in a romantic dinner or a movie or an evening at the bowling alley when your child is so sick, and the child herself might put up a fuss about it. But children are like sponges, absorbing the emotional atmosphere around them. When Mom and Dad are a strong unit, in love not just with their family but each other, the child's world, her healing space, is more stable, happier, less stressful, and so, more beneficial. Enlisting a grandparent, aunt, or uncle, or investing the time to find a good, reliable babysitter so that, every once in a while, Mom and Dad can have the uninterrupted time to refresh their connection to each other is often one of the best investments parents can make in a child's happiness.

We are used to being kind to our children. We expect it *of* ourselves. Being kind *to* ourselves is frequently something we have to learn how to do, but it, too, is a part of our child's recovery.

LAB RESULTS

Now that we've got a handle on the yeast problem, the next thing my patients' parents and I do at our second meeting is go over the results of the lab work I have ordered for their child. Because the results of each test are different for each child—sometimes in subtle ways and, at other times, more distinctly—it won't be productive to talk here about each possible variable, nor would it be a good use of space, as that would be a book unto itself. Rather, what I want to do is to tell you a little bit about the laboratory tests I usually order for each child—why I order the test and how the information that test will provide to me is important to the child's care. Though the reasons for some of these tests may not become entirely apparent to you until you have read further in this book (why I test for glutathione levels, for example), in most cases these tests are establishing baselines that the parents and I will use as a guide as the child progresses through treatment.

Complete Blood Count

A complete blood count (CBC) test is more or less exactly what it sounds like and is one of the most basic tests a physician can ask for. It measures the number of red blood cells (RBCs, which transport oxygen throughout the body) and the number of white blood cells (WBCs, which fight infection). It measures the size of the RBCs and the fraction of the blood that is composed of RBCs, which is known as *hematocrit*. And it also measures the total amount of hemoglobin in the blood; hemoglobin is the part of the RBC that transports oxygen from the lungs to wherever in the body it needs to go.

Comprehensive Metabolic Panel

A comprehensive metabolic panel (CMP) is also a standard test that doctors use as a broad screening for information about how a patient's kidneys and liver are functioning, electrolyte and acid-base balance, and blood sugar and blood proteins. This test helps doctors rule out diabetes or kidney or liver disease in the patient, and it helps us to monitor the effect any medications might have on the child's kidneys or liver.

Lipid Panel

A lipid is, in the broadest sense, merely a fat-soluble, naturally occurring molecule—fats, waxes, oils, *cholesterol*. In older people, this test lets their doctor know if they are at risk for heart attack or stroke that may be caused by a lipid-generated blockage in the blood vessels or hardening of the arteries. In my practice, I rely on this test to tell me about the child's triglycerides and cholesterol levels—high-density lipoprotein cholesterol (HDL-C, or the "good" kind), and low-density lipoprotein cholesterol (LDL-C, the "bad" kind). Your child's lipid levels may reveal more metabolic dysregulation and are important in helping to direct a healthy dietary regimen.

Erythrocyte Sedimentation Rate and High-Sensitivity C-Reactive Protein

These tests have names that aren't as straightforward sounding as the others we've just talked about, but what they do is pretty fundamental—and central: the erythrocyte sedimentation rate (ESR) is one way of assessing inflammation in the body, and the high-sensitivity C-reactive protein (CRP) measures the amount of a specific protein in the blood that alerts us to *acute* inflammation.

Stool Microbiology

I send the stool sample you will have taken from your child to a specialized lab to test for all bacteria that may be present in the stool sample, as well as to measure for yeast. These results provide us with valuable information we need to determine the integrity of the child's gut, as well as the effectiveness of certain probiotics and whether or not the dosage is sufficient.

Glutathione and Cysteine

Again, this test goes to a specialized laboratory. It tests for glutathione and cysteine levels in the child's blood. In Visit #3, we'll talk more about glutathione and its importance as an antioxidant.

RBC Elements

This is a test, once more assigned to a specialized lab, that will tell your doctor about the *intracellular* minerals and toxic elements that may be part of the composition of your child's blood. Remember that it is *inside* the cells of the body that clockwork gears spin and the work of the human body gets done. See the discussion of minerals in the next section of this chapter, Supplements.

Immunologic Evaluation

The reasons for this evaluation are fairly self-explanatory—your doctor is looking to find information on the current status of your child's immune system so that she or he can know the best avenues to take in healing it. The specific tests I ask for are IgA, IgM, and IgG, with subclasses, as well as a lymphocyte enumeration that will assess lymphocyte subsets, including natural killer cells, which are a major part of our innate immune systems and perform such vital functions as rejecting tumors and cells that are infected by viruses.

Tissue Transglutaminase IgG and IgA

Transglutaminases are a specific family of enzymes. In this test, your doctor is looking to find out if the child is suffering from celiac disease. People who suffer from celiac disease share with autistic children an intolerance for gluten.

25-OH Vitamin D₃ Level

This test measures the level of vitamin D_3 your child has at his disposal. In the next section of this chapter, Supplements, I'll talk more about how integral vitamin D_3 is to both physical and emotional well-being, and why it is an alarming trend that none of us is getting enough of it.

T4 Free, T3 Free, and Thyroid-Stimulating Hormone (TSH)

These tests refer to the thyroid gland. The work of the thyroid gland, a butterfly-shaped gland at the lower front of the neck, is to take iodine, a mineral found in many foods, and convert it to the thyroid hormones triiodothyronine (T3) and thyroxine (T4). These thyroid hormones help each cell in every organ and tissue in the body to work efficiently—brain, heart, muscle and every other organ—and they also help the body to use energy and to stay warm, so it's important to know the amount of them that is circulating in your child's system. Abnormal thyroid function tests can tell us if the gland is failing to do its job, which is a critical piece of information, as many autistic kids eventually, without intervention, develop autoimmune thyroid conditions.

Measles, Mumps, Rubella, Human Herpes Virus 6 (Roseola), and Varicella (Chicken Pox) Quantitative Titers

A titer is a measurement of the concentration of a substance in a solution, in this case the amount of antibodies to a specific disease in a child's blood. The amount of titers can tell your doctor if the child has immunity to the specific diseases he or she is testing for and be very helpful in determining the course of the medical treatment that should be provided to her.

Myelin Basic Protein Autoantibodies

This is another blood test used in checking for and monitoring diseases such as multiple sclerosis and optic neuritis. What it will tell your doctor is whether there are antibodies to myelin basic protein-producing cells at work in the child's body that might be involved in inflammatory demyelination, a condition that needs to be either ruled out or treated aggressively.

There are many other medical tests, of course, that I may order as follow-ups to this roster of what I consider the basics. The doctor's toolbox is full of them. Depending on what these basic tests tell me, I might, for instance, order a complete gut evaluation, including a comprehensive digestive stool analysis, urine peptide/opiates analysis, or a food allergy profile. I might want to know the child's serotonin level, or ask for hormone studies, including growth hormone, or a fatty acid panel. I work from the premise that the more information one has on hand, the better the decisions can be made for the child's health; but I also believe that testing, especially in the case of a disease whose treatment is as complicated as autism's, should be ongoing as the needs dictate. I either repeat testing or ask for additional tests on an average of two to three times a year, as your clinician likely will as well.

SUPPLEMENTS

Before we talk about the specific supplements your clinician is most apt to prescribe for your child, let's review some of the reasons that nutrition is so vital in the treatment of autism. The supplement schedule you and your doctor will evolve for your child will almost certainly be extensive, and perhaps complicated, with supplements in a variety of dosages that are to be given at various times in the day.

A great many people in the United States are not getting the vitamins and minerals they need to preserve optimal health. Studies have shown that almost half the population is deficient in vitamin C, for example, and over 80 percent aren't getting enough magnesium. There is very nearly a crisis in the general population concerning contemporary deficits of vitamin D, as you'll see when we discuss it in the pages to follow.

But for our children, these nutritional deficits are exacerbated in scope because of the malabsorption problems common in autistic kids. Chronic diarrhea, constipation, and intestinal inflammation reduce the amount of nutrients their systems are able to absorb. Their systems are unable to use efficiently even the smaller amounts of nutrients the general population can take away from the standard diet. Recent studies have found that autistic children measure low in levels of vitamins A, B_1, B_3, B_5, and B_{12}, calcium, selenium, zinc, and magnesium, to name but a few essential nutrients. This problem with absorption is one of the reasons I use the term *malnutrition* in association with autism.

In addition to supporting our kids' nutrient levels with supplements, however, we have to be very careful to give them the right *brands* of supplements. For example, Dr. William Walsh at Health Research Institute/Pfeiffer Treatment Center in Illinois discovered that over 99 percent of the 500 autistic children he tested had elevated serum copper to zinc ratios. The upshot of this finding is that we now know autistic kids need to avoid copper and increase their zinc intake, but most multivitamin/mineral supplements contain copper. Doctors who treat autistic kids biomedically are attuned to such nuances and will have brands of supplements to recommend that are manufactured with the special nutritional needs of autistic kids in mind.

Your child's supplement schedule is designed to compensate for the nutrients he is unable to take away from his diet alone, as well as to take into consideration his special needs, such as a copper intolerance. It will support his body in the most basic of ways—by helping to make sure his body has the tools it needs to grow, and to defend and to repair itself—and it will accomplish that most miraculous of things: it will make your child *feel better*. A child who feels better can play better, learn better, love better. The supplement schedule will be composed thoughtfully and, in the main, from the compounds I'm going to talk about now. For your most convenient reference, I've organized them alphabetically. Be strict about the schedule your doctor recommends.

5-Hydroxytryptophan

Listed first because it starts with a number, 5-hydroxytryptophan (5HTP) is an immediate precursor to serotonin. Serotonin is, in the brain, our "happy juice," and many of our children are lacking in serotonin. Where melatonin (listed with the "m" supplements), starts sleep, 5HTP helps to continue it, so on several levels, 5HTP in carefully titrated doses may be a godsend to some of our families.

Aloe Vera Juice

Yes, aloe vera juice is, indeed, the product of that beautiful house plant you probably keep around for one of its other healing properties: if you burn yourself while whipping up that delicious pork stir-fry, you can snap off a segment of the plant and apply the sap as an effective healing ointment. In its juice form, we use it for its anti-fungal properties in treating yeast infestations and to aid in relieving constipation.

Digestive Enzymes

Digestive enzymes are proteins the body manufactures, in the lining of the gut, that help it to break down food so that it can be absorbed. But autistic children, because of their gut disease, often don't naturally make enough of these digestive enzymes, especially the enzyme known as DPP–4, and thus can't break down gluten or casein, or even some of the components of foods that are GFCF diet-legal, like some carbohydrates, vegetables, and meats. Fortifying your child with supplemental digestive enzymes prior to each meal helps his body to more fully use the nutrients that are available in his foods and supplements. This helps to create a healthy digestive environment so that almost every other system and cell in his body works better too—from the immune system to neurotransmitter receptors.

Dimethylglycine

Dimethylglycine (DMG), is technically not a supplement but a food. In very small amounts, it's found in such pantry staples as brown rice—and in such kid-unfriendly items as liver. It's been sold over the counter in health food stores for years, and, in fact, the only reason it is not called a vitamin, like vitamin B, which, chemically, it resembles quite closely, is because while there are a wide range of benefits in taking it, there are no specific symptoms associated with a DMG deficiency.

We use DMG, or sometimes a close relative, TMG (trimethylglycine), in the biomedical treatment of autism as methylation support. You'll read more about methylation chemistry in Visit #3; here, let's suffice to say that within days of starting this supplement, parents have reported that their child's behavior is much improved—her eye contact is better, she is more talkative, and her tolerance level for frustration is much increased. There can be a tendency for hyperactivity or aggression with DMG or TMG; sometimes it improves spontaneously, sometimes it's managed well with careful dose titration, and sometimes it's intolerable and we just can't use it.

Essential Fatty Acids

Essential fatty acids (EFAs) are, well, just that—essential. They serve the body in a myriad of ways, but for autistic kids, it is EFAs' ability to affect mood, behavior, speech, and inflammation that is key.

What makes the EFAs essential is that the body can't construct these fats in any way at all; they can be obtained only through diet and supplements. Cod liver oil is a good supplemental source. *Cod liver oil!* I can hear any parent groaning who might once have been forced to swallow a spoonful of old-fashioned, stinky, sardine-flavored grease. Fear not! Cod liver oil is now available in chewable pills that taste, for all the world, like sugar-coated Gummi bears. Imagine kids asking for cod liver oil! It's the one supplement my patients make sure their moms and dads never run out of.

Gamma-Aminobutyric Acid

Gamma-aminobutyric acid (GABA) is the most pervasive *inhibitory* neurotransmitter in the human body. When we are excited, GABA is what helps us to settle down and relax. I use it as a calming aid for kids who are hyperactive. It also promotes speech—sometimes improving fluency, sometimes articulation, sometimes both.

L-Methylfolate

The unmethylated form of this supplement is known as folic acid, or vitamin B_9. Autistic kids can lack the functional enzymes necessary to process folic acid—to convert it to L-methylfolate—so that it can be useful to the body. In Visit #3, you'll read about how the deficit of L-methylfolate, caused by the dysfunction of the child's folate metabolism, causes one of the critical snake-eating-its-tail cycles in autistic kids. Two of the prescription-requiring supplements we use with great success to boost folate metabolism are CerefolinNAC and Deplin. Nonprescription methylfolate is also available as a supplement in lower doses.

Lysine

Lysine is an essential amino acid the body needs for a variety of functions, including repairing tissues and fighting disease. A lack of lysine has also been linked to many of the problems autistic kids suffer, including lack of concentration and irritability. Additionally, it has good antiviral properties and so is a good immune-function enhancer.

Melatonin

Melatonin is a hormone that is produced in the pineal gland, a small gland in the brain that helps to regulate circadian rhythms of sleep and wakefulness. The level of it in a healthy body will vary during the daily cycle of light and dark, as its production is partly determined by sunlight. It's become a fairly common remedy for insomnia, is used in the treatment of seasonal affective disorder (SAD), and helps blind people, who don't have day and night as a reference point, to regulate their circadian rhythms. Autistic children can frequently experience sleep difficulties, and a low dose of melatonin 20 minutes before bedtime can help to alleviate the problem.

Milk Thistle

Milk thistle is a flowering plant of the daisy family. It's been used for two thousand years to treat liver disease and to protect the liver against toxins—and it's just as useful today for the same purposes.

Minerals

There are seven *macrominerals*—calcium, magnesium, chloride, phosphorus, potassium, sodium, and sulfur—that the human body needs in significant doses in order to remain healthy. We also need *trace* amounts of a dozen other minerals, including iodine, boron, and, especially, zinc. But there are several things that can go wrong in our bodies to prevent the uptake of minerals, and—this will come as no surprise—these are among the things that go wrong in autistic bodies. Three of the minerals that autistic kids commonly require in higher doses are calcium, magnesium, and zinc.

Calcium

Most of us are familiar with the fact that a lack of calcium in our diet now will lead to osteoporosis down the road. Ninety-nine percent of the calcium in our bodies is stored in our bones and teeth—it is what supports our very structure. What may surprise you is that calcium is also necessary for the secretion of hormones and enzymes, for the efficient functioning of neurotransmitters, and for both muscle and blood vessel contraction, among the many other vital ways our bodies use the mineral.

Magnesium

Intracellular blood studies reveal that autistic children can have low levels of magnesium, a necessary mineral and one that evidence shows can have a calming effect on children with ASD.

Zinc

Zinc plays a huge part in the methylation process. We'll go into this in detail in Visit #3.

Phosphatidylcholine

Phosphatidylcholine (PC) is part of a family of compounds known as phospholipids, which are part of the makeup of cell membranes. They supply choline to the cell, which protects the cell's integrity as well as helps the cell to take nutrients in and to move toxins out. PC is especially protective of the liver, an organ that is responsible for helping to remove waste (toxins) from the body and that is particularly overburdened in autistic kids. Source is especially important with PC, and here again, most clinicians have preferred brands.

Probiotics

According to the World Health Organization (WHO), in its 2002 report "Guidelines for the Evaluation of Probiotics in Food," probiotics are defined as "Live microorganisms which when administered in adequate amounts confer a health benefit on the host." Because probiotics are one of the first supplements biomedical practitioners recommend, your child has likely been deriving the health benefits of these microorganisms for several weeks by the time of your second visit with your doctor.

Many doctors and nutritionists these days routinely recommend probiotics after a course of antibiotics to their general patient population, mostly in the form of yogurt, because antibiotics, while doing their work of killing off unwanted bacteria, also kill off the good gut flora that is necessary to maintain gut integrity. Unfortunately, autistic children usually have had more than their fair share of infections and, so, often have to take more than their fair share of antibiotics. They also can't eat yogurt, which is a dairy product and contains casein. That's where bottled probiotics come in, but make sure the brand you are buying doesn't contain any dairy. Taking nondairy, bottled probiotics helps the child's good gut flora to reestablish itself. In turn, when the gut is healthy, the immune system works better, oxidative stress is lowered, and the body's attempts to rid itself of toxins are more fruitful.

Secretin

Secretin is a peptide hormone, and its primary function in the body is to help regulate gastric acid secretion. Supplementing secretin helps to normalize the often-impaired digestive systems of autistic children. It can also help to regulate the rage center in the brain. While expensive and not effective for every child, in certain children secretin can be that silver bullet we all hope for.

Vitamins

As I said in Visit # 1, Part 1, one of the first supplements we start our kids on is a good multivitamin that is rich in B complex, so prior to reviewing the results of your child's lab work, you've already gotten a head start on this part of the program. Depending on what the laboratory reports have to say, there is a chance that your doctor will recommend boosting the intake of certain vitamins. The most common boosts we recommend are vitamin B_6, vitamin C, and vitamin D_3.

Vitamin B_6

Vitamin B_6 helps to maintain blood sugar, or glucose, within a normal range; it is what your body needs to make hemoglobin—the part of the blood that carries oxygen throughout your body; and it helps with the functioning of both the nervous system and the immune system. Of particular importance to autistic children, vitamin B_6 works with digestive enzymes to metabolize proteins so that nutrients can be absorbed and used by the body and leaky guts can heal. Vitamin B_6 has also been shown to help in controlling certain seizures; for this reason, it can play a huge role in managing that particular problem.

Vitamin C
Vitamin C, found in many foods, particularly citrus fruits, is a natural antioxidant and, as such, is also a natural chelator. Among the critical functions it helps the body to perform are helping the immune system to manage infections; helping the body to form collagen, a protein used to make skin, blood vessels, tendons, ligaments, and, when the body is injured, scar tissue; and healing wounds. For autistic kids, who often have low levels of it, vitamin C can also help to calm stereotypical behaviors because of the way it influences the brain's response to the neurotransmitter dopamine.

Vitamin D$_3$
How shall I begin to extol the benefits of vitamin D$_3$ supplements?

For over a hundred years, science has recognized the importance of this vitamin in developing and maintaining healthy bones, but as more research is conducted, we are discovering that a lack of vitamin D$_3$ is also a significant factor in all sorts of other diseases and conditions. Vitamin D$_3$ has been linked to the relief of back pain; to the treatment of high blood pressure, diabetes, multiple sclerosis, and rheumatoid arthritis; to fending off an insulin resistance during pregnancy; and to increasing the efficacy of the immune system. It's also been suggested that it can help to protect against cancer. Vitamin D$_3$, you see, is the only vitamin that can be taken into the body transdermally, through the rays of the sun; as long ago as the 1940s, researchers were noticing that people who lived in sunny latitudes had a reduced rate of death from cancer and speculated that it was because of the vitamin D$_3$ they were receiving from the sunlight.

Today, unfortunately, most people don't spend a lot of time in the sun. This is partially because our lifestyles don't require that most of us spend our days in the fields plowing and harvesting. It is also because, when we do go outside, the fear of skin cancer has led us all to slather ourselves in ultraviolet (UV) protection; our sunscreens do indeed keep us from getting burned, but excessive use of them every time we step outdoors also blocks our body's ability to receive the supply of vitamin D_3 we were meant to get from the sun. Even folks who already take a supplemental form of vitamin D_3 are likely to be basing their dosage on recommendations that are outdated—200 IU a day until age 50, and, after that, 400 IU a day; many prominent researchers today are saying that doses of 2,000–4,000 IU are more in line with what we now know the body needs, with 10,000 IU a day being the upper limit of what may cross the line into too much vitamin D_3.

None of us are getting enough of the stuff, and this lack has a more significant impact upon autistic kids, with their less hearty physical systems, than it does on most of the rest of us. Two areas that vitamin D_3 impacts are of particular concern as they apply to autism. The first is vitamin D_3's influence on cognitive function. Scientists are finding a positive correlation between levels of this vitamin and performance on mental function tests.

The second area of concern is depression. In one study of older adults, vitamin D_3 deficiency was linked to not only low cognition, but also low mood. Autistic kids can suffer from bad moods, and a lot of those kids are on mood-enhancing pharmaceuticals as a result. In my practice, while I'm not averse to mood-enhancing pharmaceuticals and will certainly turn to their use when I think it's warranted, I'd much rather start an ill-tempered child on gradually increasing doses of vitamin D_3 and see if that gets us where we want to go without having to put one more chemical into his system.

How does vitamin D_3 work to enhance mood?

Okay, picture a room—living room, bedroom, any old room will do. On one wall of the room is a window, and on the opposite wall there's a door. The door and window are there and are open because this room is meant to be filled with a constant flow of water, and they are what maintain the water level, with the water coming into the room through the window and flowing out through the door. The water flow is controlled by how far the window and the door happen to be open.

When the door and the window are both wide open, the water flows freely, and the level in the room stays constant, say at between three and five feet, enough to splash around in and swim. But when the window is closed, very little water flows in, but plenty continues to flow out, so the water level can go down to just a few soggy inches.

Now, picture yourself in this room, and pretend that your whole job in life is to swim in it. When the water level is at three feet, you can splash around a little—swimming at that level may not be much fun, but you can do it. When the water is at five feet, man, you can do laps and somersaults and really have a grand old time, so your work of swimming seems more like play.

Biochemically, the amount of water in our metaphorical room is determined by how much serotonin is available to our brain. Our body can produce some of it, allowing us three feet of water in which to plod through, or it can produce a greater amount, which allows us five feet of water and a lot of fun. The amount of serotonin our bodies are able to manufacture is key to determining our mood—whether we plod through life or whether we have a lot of fun with it.

Pharmaceutical mood enhancers work by closing the door to our room so that the water can't flow out; the trickle that comes in is collected, and the water level eventually stabilizes—that is, in effect, trapping the serotonin the body does manufacture. But this presumes the window is open and something is coming in through it. If this is not the case, something we find frequently in our children with autism, then closing the door may prove not only futile, but counterproductive.

What opens the window? Vitamin D_3.

When we don't get enough vitamin D_3, our room fills with only inches of water, in which we can do no more than get our feet wet, so our job of swimming is a sad, crashing bore.

Vitamin D_3, by opening the window, enables the body to produce its own, natural serotonin from 5HTP, and, in consequence, it enables the natural flow of the water—the natural and proper bio-chemistry—to both continue and stabilize. The job of swimming—the job of living life—becomes pleasant, and even joyous.

And, after all, this is why we are going through this process at all—joy. We are doing all this work to regain for our child the joy of living, and for ourselves the joy of seeing our child growing up healthy and happy.

VISIT #2

ACTION LIST

Begin the yeast detoxification process.
This includes changing your child's diet to minimize sugars and glycemic carbohydrates. It may include the use of a prescription antifungal. Watch your child carefully so that you're ready to help her through this process by cutting back on the antifungal drugs, adding activated charcoal or aloe juice to her supplement schedule, and drawing warm, Epsom salt baths when necessary to ease the discomfort of yeast die-off.

Be strict about your supplement schedule.
You and your clinician have in all likelihood customized the partial list of supplements I've outlined in this chapter to fit your child's particular profile of nutrient needs. Because your child's supplement schedule is customized, there is, alas, no standard chart that is available to you to, say, simply print out from an Internet website and follow with confidence that you are doing all, or even the best, required for your child's recovery. My advice is to make your own chart based on the decisions you and your doctor make together for your child.

Some parents maintain the chart on a computerized spreadsheet. They list the supplements in one column, the dosages in another, the time of day in a third, the dates in a fourth, and so on. This can be a good method; if you leave room for a final column in which to record your child's response to each supplement, this spreadsheet style can be a very precise augmentation of your recovery diary.

Speaking of precision, when I say be strict, I mean make sure you get your supplements in. If your multivitamin is to be given twice daily, give it twice daily. You do not have to give it at 8:27 AM and 7:34 PM, just give it in the morning and in the evening. Enzymes should ideally be given 20–30 minutes before all meals. Dani wouldn't get lunch if she had to go to the nurse's office at school to get enzymes, so we don't try. And my approach at home is much less Martha Stewart precise and far more June Cleaver complete: enzymes are often chucked down the hatch just as we pray, and I offer an extra prayer that the best I can do will be good enough.

When our family embarked on Dani's recovery, my own method was to handwrite the list and post it on the inside of the cupboard door where the supplements were kept, changing it out whenever the supplement schedule needed to be updated. This far less technical method worked out just fine, and it's a method we still use, but with a twist. As Dani got better, she started to take some interest in drawing or coloring, and one of the tasks she assigned herself was to make up her own supplement chart. At first, I noted each of the pertinent pieces of information on the chart, but she decorated it whimsically with flowers and butterflies, or portraits of her favorite football players, depending on her mood when it was time to update the chart. Now, let me tell you that when Dani began taking the array of supplements that is required to support her illness—and taking them twice a day—the process irritated her, and she would sometimes resist. But in the simple act of decorating the chart, the chart became hers. She became invested in following the plan that she herself had had a part in making up. Now, as she's grown older and recovered so much cognitive function, I direct her about specific supplements and dosages, but she creates the chart herself, staying invested, and learning to take responsibility for her own supplement schedule.

Keep your recovery diary up-to-date.
Now that you are beginning to kill yeast and to support your child's system with a full range of supplements, the changes in physical and behavioral symptoms may start to happen at a swifter pace, both in a positive way and as regression as yeast die-off happens or a supplement is not tolerated. Your record of these changes, both the spectacular and the more subtle ones, will be a chief resource in your child's ongoing care.

JEDI KNIGHTS, YODA, AND GLUTATHIONE

DEFINING PROGRESS

Through the course of our lives, all of us encounter defining moments—those events that irrevocably sever the lives we had been living from the lives we will, forever forward, lead. These events can be the historic crises we use to collectively date our trajectories: Where were you when JFK was shot? When the *Challenger* exploded? When the twin towers fell? They can be very personal, and joyous—graduation from high school or college, or your wedding day; and they can also be tragic—the death of a parent, or the diagnosis of your child's disease.

In the days before my daughter's diagnosis, I was, as I said, a typical pediatrician taking care of mostly well children; in the days since, I have become an expert on the treatment of autism. Now, the priorities in my home have changed. They revolve, like yours, around the management of my daughter's illness. Probably also like yours, they are tucked around the demands of full-time work—in my case, the hectic schedule I keep to help other families manage their kids' illness too. Now, my whole family is much more appreciative of the simpler pleasures—a day spent cheering at a football game, an evening spent in the company of my son at one of his Boy Scout events, the peace of singing in the church choir, or even just the comfort of being all together. Now, I travel the world giving lectures and teaching other doctors about the biomedical approach to ASD. Now, too, I mentor those physicians who come to me to spend the days and weeks and months in my office that it will take for them to become experts in biomedical intervention.

Bill Smithfield is one of the doctors who is learning with me to be an autism specialist. His motivation? His son is one of the one-in-six kids who have recently been diagnosed with ASD. As it is in my case, it frequently happens that doctors who choose to train in my specialty have a vested interest in it. The way a medical researcher might decide to devote his career to the study of breast cancer because his mother suffered with it, many ASD specialists are born because of the defining moment of an ASD diagnosis in their own families. It is fairly natural to be directed in life by our own defining moments—and it is why those of us who work with autistic kids frequently bring our defining moments, and the empathy and passion they create, to our work. The doctors who train with me are, simply, passionate about gaining the tools that will help them to help others.

This is why, on his second visit to my office, I think Bill was more than a little disappointed when he walked in the door that morning. You see, in transforming my practice from a typical pediatric office to one that specializes in autism, I had retained all my previous patients. Frequently, in between seeing my autistic patients, I'll have an appointment with a teenage girl who's been under my care since she was an infant, and now she's due for her standard annual physical; or with a little boy who merely needs to have a wart removed from his knee. The second morning that Bill walked into my office, my waiting room seemed to be filled with these sorts of typical patients.

"No autism cases this morning, Julie?" he asked, a reasonable question considering his need and desire to learn, not to mention the fact that the drive from his home to my office was quite a long one. There was no reason for him to be here if we weren't going to be talking biomedical protocol; he already knew all about standard annual physicals and wart removal. But I just smiled. What Bill was seeing in my waiting room of typically rambunctious kids at play was clear-cut evidence of the efficacy of biomedical intervention: he couldn't tell, after the cursory glance he gave them as he walked through the lobby, the autistic kids from the typical ones.

By now, by your third visit to your autism specialist, you should be able to see such evidence for yourself, in your own child. You have changed her diet to *remove* the gluten and casein that upset her delicate digestive system. You have fortified her cellular strength by adding vitamins, minerals, enzymes, and probiotic supplements that *replenish* those critical elements of human biochemistry that she either lacked or had been unable to properly digest. By killing yeast you have begun to *repair* some of the damage she has sustained, and, through all these efforts, you have begun to *restore* normal GI and immune system function.

You, of course, can't see her molecular structure. You can't see her cells growing stronger and stronger and the vicious, dysfunctional cycles being broken. How can you tell if the clockwork gears are beginning to mesh seamlessly again? What are some of the signs of progress you will likely have noted in your child's recovery diary?

- Her stools are definitely better. Sometimes they are still "soft-serve-like," but they are not explosive, and they happen on a much more regular schedule.
- His eye contact is better. He looks straight at you when he informs you, "No!"—and he finds your face and holds it in his gaze when he wants a hug.
- She is starting to generate word approximations. She is likely speaking more, and her language is clearer and more easily understandable.

- His tantrums are remarkably improved. He is pitching way fewer fits, the ones he does indulge in are less intense and of a shorter duration, and he allows you to console him.
- Her appetite is improving. Her cravings are subsiding and she is amenable to trying new foods.
- He just seems happier in the skin he is in—the underlying discomfort and infernal itch are abating.
- Oh, and by the way? She hasn't been sick with a cold or a sinus infection or an earache in nearly two months!

Remember that every child is unique, because every person's biochemistry is unique; these are examples of typical recovery milestones for you to use as a guideline, but they may not fit your own child's case exactly. The point is, you will be starting to see the hard work you are doing—and the harder work you child is doing—reap rewards. What is the next step? What is the next thing you want to incorporate into your child's routine on the way to recovery?

THE NEXT LEVEL

When you started your first real job—and by that I don't mean the paper route you had when you were a kid, but the first entry-level position you took that launched you on your career trajectory—you knew that you were expected to perform certain tasks and meet certain goals and that when you did those things, you were likely going to be rewarded with some tangible advancement for your efforts.

When you decided to get serious about your physical fitness, and resolved to turn in your couch potato ID card, you didn't—if you were smart—go to the gym on the first day and put in five miles on the treadmill or do a full set of bicep curls with 20-pound weights. You started slow and graduated to longer runs and heavier dumbbells.

Possibly the most graphic experience of moving from one level to another is those video games your kids play. When they satisfactorily complete all the tasks required at the first level—say, blowing up enough enemy starships in the allotted time—bells ring, whistles blow, neonlike screens flash, and they are invited to play at the next, more advanced level.

That may seem as if it is exactly what you have been doing in your biomedical program—advancing in an orderly fashion from one level to the next—and in many ways, it is simply a matter of taking one careful step after another. I'll caution you once again, however, that as you take each progressive step along the biomedical path, your child may show signs of improvement more quickly than you could ever have hoped, then regress suddenly, then improve again just as suddenly as you vary the dosage of his supplements or discover another troublesome food and remove it from his diet. But your goal is always to keep strengthening and normalizing your child's systems toward a slow and steady advancement to the next level.

The concept of advancement—whether it is career advancement, a harder workout at the gym, or getting really, *really* good at *Call of Duty*—is almost always the result of a number of interdependent processes working in harmony. You probably won't get that next big promotion at work, for example, if your ability to multitask like Angelina Jolie is your only talent. That one skill needs to be complemented by polished organizational, interpersonal, and leadership skills. At the gym, you'll combine an aerobic workout with weight-bearing and stretching exercises to achieve optimal fitness. Getting really, *really* good at *Call of Duty* involves not only understanding the rules of a complex game but also honing the eye-hand coordination required to play it.

I'm stressing this concept of advancement as the result of the harmonious meshing of acquired skills and knowledge because it applies to all our attempts to get good at anything in life—at our jobs, at our play, or at managing our health and that of our sick kids. As we discuss the next level of biomedical treatment, I want you to think of the complex and interdependent biochemical processes we're about to talk about—sulfation and methylation chemistries, folate metabolism, and glutathione production—in the same terms: each of these is an independent biological process, but unless all of them are working efficiently, none of them will work very well at all.

SULFATION

One of the leading researchers in the biochemistry of autism, Rosemary Waring, has conducted numerous studies that show 73–92 percent of children with ASD have impaired sulfation chemistry—that is, they have low plasma sulfate levels. The urine of children with autism has been found to contain almost twice the amount of sulfate as that of typical children in a control group—meaning that autistic children have only about one-fifth the normal level of sulfate their systems need to work.

What this means on a chemical level is that because they lack sulfur, they may have trouble processing *phenols,* which are chemicals found in nearly all food groups. The good news is that you have already assisted your child's body in starting to solve this problem because chemical phenols are often a part of artificial food ingredients, and on the GFCF diet, your child is no longer eating very much artificial, or junk, food.

But phenols are also found in naturally healthy foods such as fruits and vegetables and in *phenolic amines* such as serotonin and dopamine, which are critical neurotransmitters. Clearly, removing phenols from your child's diet, as you have removed gluten and casein, is not a viable option for most families, and is unnecessary for the vast majority of us. This is fortunate, because removing phenols in addition to gluten and casein from your child's diet starts to feel like the "Air" diet. While certain to give them nothing harmful, consuming only air is unpopular with most children and parents, and is not nutritionally sound. So instead of completely removing phenols, you need to help your child to better process the ones she eats.

Well, that's easy, right? You need to augment her sulfation pathways in some way.

Right. But let's talk first about the larger biological ramifications of low sulfur and how they relate specifically to autism. As we do this, keep in mind that our goal here is not to be comprehensive, but only to teach a concept with a couple of examples so that the rationale for fixing things such as sulfation in your child makes sense to you.

Phenols are processed by the enzyme phenol sulfotransferase (PST). PST is produced in the body through the oxidation of sulfur-containing foods. Children with low sulfate levels don't have the sulfur they need to produce, or produce enough, PST. This condition, called both phenol intolerance and faulty sulfation, degrades the body's ability to detoxify itself. It interferes with the elimination of heavy metals. It compromises digestion and gut integrity. And it impairs the body's clockwork gears, disrupting cellular activity at the molecular level. In short, it impacts nearly every physiologic function associated with a diagnosis of autism—and it causes a whole menu of signs and symptoms, many of which are classic to a diagnosis of autism and other ASDs:

- hyperactivity
- impaired neuromolecular function
- self-injurious behavior
- headaches
- reddened cheeks or ears
- inappropriate laughter
- irritability and impatience
- poor sleep habits
- aggression and tantrum throwing
- diarrhea
- mental fog.

As another example of the impact of sulfur on our metabolic clockwork gears, the body needs sulfur to produce the hormone cholecystokinin (CCK). CCK stimulates the release of oxytocin, a neurotransmitter that is critical to socialization and that is found in low levels in autistic kids. With more study, we may find that it is this inability to efficiently manufacture and utilize oxytocin that helps to explain some of the antisocial behavior related to autism.

Although there is, currently, no reliable and widely and commercially available test that will directly determine a child's degree of sulfation dysfunction, and the cognitive or behavioral clues might be very subtle, you might think back to how your child has reacted in the past to eating (or even craving) foods that have a high content of natural *salicylates* (a subgroup of phenols), such as grapes or apples, or ingesting heavy chemical phenols of the kind contained in Tylenol, or snacking on foods with artificial ingredients. In some cases, the child may be so sensitive to phenols that the signs and symptoms she has ingested them will begin to show as soon as 20 minutes after eating.

All right, now that we know the problem, how do we help to fix it? Fortunately, there are any number of ways to increase sulfur levels.

One simple solution to replacing sulfur in the body is through regular soaks in Epsom salt baths, and there are sulfate creams now available that also convey sulfur into the system transdermally. And—more good news—you are likely already giving your child more of the vitamins and minerals that help to support the sulfation process, notably, magnesium and folate.

A diet rich in folate, also known as vitamin B_9, is, of course, the optimal way to meet the body's need. Dark, leafy greens such as kale and spinach, brussels sprouts, beets, turnips, and avocados all contain high amounts of folate, though as both a mother and a pediatrician, I'm realistic about the foods we can actually get our children to willingly move from their plates to their mouths. In our house, we've had success in adapting some of the recipes in Jessica Seinfeld's cookbook *Deceptively Delicious* for the GFCF diet—basically hiding nutrient-rich foods that kids are known to reject within recipes for foods they will readily eat. Spinach in tomato sauces for rice pasta and cabbage in cakes—that sort of thing has proven to be quite effective. If you are a home cook, it's a strategy I can recommend.

But why is folate so important to sulfation? Well, remember how I just went out of my way to stress the complex, interdependent nature of biochemical processes? Folate-rich foods and supplements boost the body's folate metabolism; normal folate metabolism triggers the body's production of *methyl-B$_{12}$* which, in turn, triggers sulfation.

METHYLATION

Follow me: chemically, folate metabolism transfers carbon units called *methyl groups* from molecule to molecule inside a cell. Methylation is the process of transferring a methyl group from one molecule to another. Basically, a methyl group consists of one carbon atom with four little "sticky spots." Three of the sticky spots are paired with hydrogen atoms, and the fourth is always either looking for a date, or ready to dump the date it has and pick up someone new. That's an inelegant comparison and, yet, apt, because the methyl group is essentially promiscuous, constantly changing out that fourth partner for the next best thing to come along. In folate metabolism, the methyl group is always switching back and forth between folate and the vitamin B$_{12}$ we eat. With inadequate folate metabolism, however, the methyl group turns into the biological equivalent of the guy who can't get the girl. As a result, the body—a body that may have a great folate and B$_{12}$ supply—simply cannot use the components it does have to get the girl and make *methyl-B$_{12}$*. Without *methyl-B$_{12}$*, sulfation doesn't happen—not to mention that brain function and detoxification, as well as reproductive function, DNA synthesis and repair, and the rate of aging are all impacted negatively.

We'll talk in more detail about how detoxification is disrupted by the dysfunction of all these processes in a few pages. Right now, I want to elaborate on what I meant by "brain dysfunction" in the last paragraph. What, exactly, happens to a brain in a body that can't produce methyl-B_{12}?

Well, myelination—the growth of the brain's white matter—is stunted. The pruning of this white matter—the configuring of it that, as we talked about earlier, makes a human brain essentially a construction zone for the first 20 or more years of life—is compromised. The formation of critical neurotransmitters such as melatonin, serotonin, creatine, and phospholipids is impeded. That's what happens. The project in the construction zone gets scrapped for lack of raw materials. The brain doesn't get built.

The mental handicaps we create by refusing to address the biochemical deficiencies of folate metabolism and sulfation and methylation chemistries in our autistic kids cannot be overstated. Denying biomedical intervention as a primary tool for fighting autism is essentially denying the potential to normalize compromised brain structure and, so, brain function.

Let's make no mistake about this: autistic kids have brain cells in as much abundance as any other kid. The cells just can't work like any other kid's. And this is the heart of the biomedical goal: to normalize what already exists so that it can work.

METHYL-B_{12}

One of the chemical components an actual working brain can take for granted, as we've noted in the last section, is methyl-B_{12}. Because autistic kids are often lacking the ability to complete the manufacture of methyl-B_{12} on their own, the next step in the biomedical approach is to furnish it to them.

Methyl-B_{12} therapy has been hailed by autism advocacy groups and autism specialists as one of the most significant treatments in the biomedical toolbox. Some doctors have reported up to a 94 percent response rate by the patients in their individual practices. Cognitive function, eye contact, initiation of interactive play, the ability to feel and interpret emotion, and even spontaneous language recovery, including increased vocabulary and the use of complex sentences—all these things may miraculously improve in patients who begin methyl-B_{12} therapy. One day a child could not talk, and then he started methyl-B_{12} therapy and he could! Stories such as this abound and are the reason I teach parents to call methyl-B_{12} simply "word vitamins."

You see, for all of the truly amazing recovery stories, methyl-B_{12} therapy does not routinely make for the instantaneous miracles with which it is often credited. In best-case scenarios, when a child loses his diagnosis of autism, that is, regains lost vocabulary and social skills and alters the other behaviors typically associated with the diagnosis, that child has usually been on the therapy for several years. It's true that even for children who make only slight or moderate improvement with the therapy, the nature of the impact is so profound that her parents more often than not opt to continue the therapy. Still, the therapy does not work for everyone, and there can be side effects.

The common side effects of methyl-B_{12} therapy include increased hyperactivity, the possibility of increased stimming, and disruption of sleep patterns. These side effects can feel a whole lot like regression to parents who have worked so diligently to this point, changing their child's diet, getting yeast infestations under control, and maintaining a complicated supplement routine. If a child whose stimming, for instance, had disappeared begins spinning in circles again, it can be disheartening. Maddening!

So let's talk about why these particular side effects may occur. We deduce this from the explanations some children are able to offer as they recover enough to try to explain what they are feeling. Let's say that you have spent your whole life wearing a pair of heavy leather gloves. I mean that you have worn these gloves every day and every night from the time when your memory begins; you don't know what it's like for your hands to feel any other way than too warm and stuffy, or to function other than clumsily, and it would never even occur to you to wonder about these things because you have never experienced any other way for your hands to be.

Then, one day, someone comes along and says, "Oh, my, it's much too hot today for you to be wearing gloves," and she shows you how to take them off.

At first your hands feel vulnerable without the gloves. You're used to having them covered, and no mater how uncomfortable that was, it was a form of protection. Now your hands feel cool, and you can stretch your fingers, and you have to become accustomed to that freedom before you can take any pleasure in it.

Ah! But soon you do begin to take pleasure in being ungloved! Every new sensation seems a thrill—the refreshing flow of water on your bare skin, the hardness and density of a baseball in your hand, and the incredible softness of a flower or a strand of a doll's silky hair between your fingertips. You take so much pleasure in each new sensation you become greedy for it, testing water temperatures and pressures under the faucet, running your palms over flower petals in the garden, and plunging your hands into its crumbling, moist earth, touching fabrics and your dog's fur and your loved ones' faces—touching, touching, touching!

For autistic kids, methyl-B_{12} therapy may feel like taking the gloves off their brains. Suddenly, they are aware of all the occasions around them for stimulation. They begin to experience all the sensations of the world—they begin to *want* to experience the sensations—but they don't yet know how to process the stimuli. They become greedy about their new awareness, absorbing their new reality eagerly and, in consequence, not always reacting appropriately to the new wonders until they learn how to cope with them.

For most children, learning how to cope with the new stimuli may take from a couple of days or weeks to as long as several months. If your child is experiencing side effects, your clinician may make adjustments in your child's dosage of methyl-B_{12}, tailoring it to the amount of methyl-B_{12} his unique systems can handle. Sadly, for a small percentage of children, the hyperactivity is so severe that they cannot tolerate any dose at all.

Fortunately, because methyl-B_{12} helps the body to manufacture melatonin, a biochemical often recommended to those who suffer from insomnia, sleep disturbances are often easily overcome, because the child begins to manufacture his own melatonin once again.

For these reasons, it's imperative that your child's diet and supplement program is stable and that it remains unchanged for at least the first few days to weeks from the start of methyl-B_{12} therapy, depending on the response of each individual child. To know if the therapy is working for your child and to adjust the dosage so that the therapy has the best chance for a positive outcome, you can't risk mixing up the causes of any unusual signs and symptoms. If your child is, for example, irritable during the first stages of methyl-B_{12} therapy, you want to know it's because of how the methyl-B_{12} is affecting her and not because she "accidentally" ate a gluten-filled cupcake for an after-school snack at a friend's house.

You will intuitively understand that this is a good approach for most of the changes introduced to our children—one thing at a time from a small dose initially, raising it to best dose for each child individually, is usually the best way to know which things are helpful and which are not. It is important to reiterate that we rarely find a "silver bullet," that one thing that "cures" the autism. Rather, it is the cumulative, additive effect of working on several of those clockwork gears simultaneously that makes for recovery.

There is one final drawback to methyl-B_{12} therapy, and it is almost always a drawback that the parents, rather than the afflicted child, have a bit of trouble facing: methyl-B_{12} is most effective when administered by subcutaneous injection. This means a shot just under the skin. The idea of giving their child a shot three or four times a week is something that often makes parents cringe.

Now, there are other ways to deliver methyl-B_{12} into the child's system. But it's critical to remember two things: (1) methyl-B_{12} is a very large molecule that does not cross easily from outside the body to inside; (2) with that problem in methylating vitamin B_{12}, our children's needs for methyl-B_{12} are exceptional. That being said, it does come in different forms. You can buy methyl-B_{12} in a pill to be given *orally*, which the child would take as part of his daily supplement routine. But remember that our children often have gut problems; the amount of the methyl-B_{12} their digestive systems can absorb is therefore limited, and the results of the therapy can, in turn, be limited too with oral dosing. There is an intranasal spray form of methyl-B_{12} that some patients use successfully. It requires, however, willingness and ability to inhale it in concert with the actual mist release. Methyl-B_{12} comes in a form meant to be taken *sublingually*—meaning, held under the tongue until it is thoroughly dissolved; but most doctors have found that few children, autistic or typical, have the patience to hold a tablet under their tongue for the length of time it takes to deliver a full dose in that manner and will end up swallowing it, so it becomes, in essence, an oral dose anyway. A hypodermic injection could also be delivered *intramuscularly*—which means a shot that penetrates more deeply than just under the skin, into muscle tissue—but tests have shown that methyl-B_{12} delivered in this manner is eliminated too quickly for the body to benefit from the full dose. Finally, methyl-B_{12} comes in creams to be delivered *transdermally*, or through the skin; theoretically, these creams should work just as well as a subcutaneous injection, but test results have shown that they don't. For the most efficacious delivery of methyl-B_{12}, nothing works better than a shallow shot in the butt.

For parents who remain squeamish about the shot, there is a device called a *shot blocker*, whose design (the bottom looks like the soles of a pair of golf shoes) distracts the child's tactile experience so that the shot's delivery is masked, and some parents use it with great success. There are also prescription creams, each with potential side effects, that can be applied prior to the injection that help to numb the skin and make the actual insertion of the needle less of an issue. But once a parent becomes comfortable and begins methyl-B$_{12}$ therapy, what he is likely to find is that the children become comfortable with it too, making the added equipment or creams unnecessary. The reason kids become comfortable with it? Well, initially, because the shot doesn't really hurt—it's always the *idea* of a shot that is more daunting than the real thing. Once a child has received a few of them, with the extremely slender needles used in methyl-B$_{12}$ therapy, receiving them regularly becomes no big deal.

But the real reason the kids come to not mind the shots is more profound: the child feels better afterward. You may find that your child, when the therapy has been ongoing for several weeks or a month, will, as many of the children in my practice do, start to *ask* for his or her shot. The momentary pinprick of the needle becomes nothing to them in comparison to all they can feel when the gloves are off and all they can say when the words are freed.

GLUTATHIONE

Now we come to the last piece of the puzzle we are tying to put together in this chapter—glutathione, that antioxidant I mentioned way back in Visit #1, Part 1 and asked you to remember. Glutathione is the body's master antioxidant. I often use my *Star Wars* analogy to explain its primacy in the scheme of human biochemistry: other antioxidants that the body produces or consumes are all noble Jedi Knights—but glutathione is Yoda. And Yoda, as we movie lovers all know, can do wondrous things.

The sulfur group that makes up glutathione has the unique capacity to bind to it mercury, lead, cadmium, arsenic, tin, nickel, and other heavy metals and toxins and remove them from the body—that is, glutathione plays an irreplaceable role in detoxification. It does this by, quite literally, capturing the molecules of heavy metals and surrounding them, then ushering them out of the body in the form of pee and poop. Glutathione is the reason that normally healthy people who like to eat a nice piece of salmon once a week don't end up with mercury poisoning. If you overtax the capacity of your glutathione reserves, however, by indulging in sushi six or seven times a week—or if you just happen to be as susceptible to environmental toxins as autistic kids are—then even Yoda will fail to get the job done.

How does the body make glutathione? Only methyl-B_{12} can activate methionine synthase's role in what is known as the methionine/homocysteine recycling pathway. And it is only this pathway that is able to activate the entire body's sulfur-based detoxification system. Only this pathway can activate the formation of S-adenosylmethionine (also known as SAMe), which is the universal methyl donor—or "date," to refer back to our previous methyl group analogy. Only through this pathway can glutathione be formed.

But your child's folate metabolism and sulfation and methylation chemistries are not allowing her to manufacture her own glutathione—so we help her with that. In this case, with glutathione *infusions.*

These infusions are simply IV (intravenous) drips, containing a formula of glutathione as well as other antioxidants such as vitamin C and, sometimes, N-acetylcysteine. The formulas are often customized for each child according to his weight and the severity of distress. It takes approximately 20 minutes for a full dose to be administered. In my office, the child spends this time sitting in a big easy chair, often cuddled in the lap of a parent or one of my staff, quietly reading a book or doing homework.

Yes, most children balk the first time or two that they are given a glutathione drip. Some do worse than balk. But in all my now-vast experience, I have yet to meet a child who didn't start to feel so much better after a series of infusions that he didn't offer up his own arm (even though he might be saying, "No, Dr. Buckley," as he does it) the moment he walked through my door on infusion day. In fact, the room set aside in my office for drawing blood and giving infusions is quite a popular place, and the kids who are waiting for their own treatments frequently pop in to see what's going on and find out if it's their turn yet. Now, for some folks, infusions just aren't feasible or logistically possible. We do *nebulize* glutathione, much like a breathing treatment for an asthmatic, and there are transdermal creams as well. But much like the methyl-B_{12} shots, those infusions of Jedi Knights and Yoda are often unparalleled for helping along the road to recovery.

One final thought on raising glutathione levels: OSR #1™. OSR was developed by Dr. Boyd Haley, a brilliant and fiercely ethical chemist who spent most of his career as the chairman of the Department of Chemistry at the University of Kentucky. It is the first of a new generation of antioxidants. Still in trials and early use as I write, this new supplement is proving to be exceptionally safe and is raising glutathione levels more effectively than we have ever before seen in medicine. As we learn that raising glutathione levels is helpful in treating so many disease processes, I suspect OSR may radically change the way we think about detoxification and disease management

THE IRONIC CYCLE

Now we know that without efficient folate metabolism and wide-open sulfation and methylation pathways, the body's ability to produce glutathione is severely curtailed. No glutathione, no heavy metal detoxification. Mercury, lead, arsenic, and other heavy metals remain lodged in the child's system, continuing to do their dirty work and, eventually, inflicting long-term and sometimes permanent damage.

But what is it that causes folate metabolism and sulfation and methylation chemistries to malfunction in the first place?

Hold on to your hat.

It is well documented in the medical literature that these metabolic processes can be disrupted from their normal function by mercury, lead, arsenic, and other heavy metals.

Yes, that's right. In other words, if you are overloaded with heavy metals that have entered your body systematically through environmental exposure, ingestion, or injection, it is those same heavy metals that shut down the very biochemical reactions that are designed to eliminate them.

It becomes another snake-eating-its-tail cycle that must be broken.

We break it by increasing the amount of sulfur in the child's system with Epsom salt baths and transdermal sulfur creams. By providing foods rich in folate or folate supplements. By methyl-B_{12} therapy and glutathione infusions. That is, we give each of the child's systems what the heavy metals are now preventing them from getting naturally. We address each of the independent processes so that the system as a whole can heal and the child's recovery can advance.

ACTION LIST

Record your child's progress.
Refer to the list that starts on page 63 and make a note each time your child reaches another milestone, large or small, along the path of recovery. Please note, as well, that treatment of autism is an evolving science and that this list is a starting point; your child may experience a symptom or symptoms that are not on this list. For the most up-to-date, comprehensive list available, please go to www. healingourautisticchildren.com.

Stabilize your child's diet and supplement routine, particularly regarding recommended dosages of magnesium and folate—supplements that help to heal dysfunctional sulfation metabolism—in preparation to beginning methyl-B$_{12}$ injections.
If your child will eat them, increase the folate-rich foods you serve to her.

Draw your child plenty of warm baths, adding one-half to one full cup of Epsom salt to the tub.
Put lots of toys in the tub and let him play in there until his fingers pucker. You may, additionally, opt to use a transdermal sulfur cream

to further increase his body's sulfur content. Drinking that bath water can cause diarrhea, so be careful, and if the skin begins to seem dry, adding some baking soda to the tub can help to offset the drying effect.

Start methyl-B$_{12}$ therapy.

Learn from your clinician the proper way to administer the subcutaneous shots. They usually come from compounding pharmacies in tiny syringes with very tiny needles, all ready to go. The shots are frequently prescribed to be given once every two to three days; your physician will determine the most appropriate initial dosage, and then you will monitor your child closely to determine whether the dosage must be adjusted. Keep detailed records of the changes you see at home and call your doctor's office if there are any problems during this process, especially during the first several weeks as your child's metaphorical gloves come off and he begins to experience all the wonders of the world that had previously been closed to him.

Schedule regular nights together as a family.

As your child adjusts to the methyl-B$_{12}$ therapy and begins to experience unaccustomed stimuli, she will benefit from and may actually participate in an extra dose of family time. Watch a good DVD together, play board games, put together a jigsaw puzzle. Try to incorporate some time just for talk, perhaps using a little game I call "I Love You Today Because . . ." to loosen things up. In the game, every family member answers that question for every other family member. The answers can range from the silly ("What I love best about you today, Mom, is you didn't wear that stupid hat again when you dropped me off at school even though it was raining") to the sublime, but the exercise can strengthen your whole family dynamic as each member verbalizes appreciation for the others.

The primary goal of the exercise, however, is to help your autistic child feel loved and accepted as he negotiates a world filled with unaccustomed sensations—and sharp new emotions—even as he sometimes reacts inappropriately to the new stimuli. Remember that even if your child can't fully participate in all of these activities yet, getting him to try to do so in small doses and letting him know that you welcome his effort is three-quarters of the battle. You'll be surprised at how he will manage to insert himself into family activities!

If recommended and feasible, schedule your first series of glutathione infusions.

Brace yourself if you need to—the first time a child is given an IV drip can feel like an endurance test. Know that you are helping her to heal by standing firm, and take your cues from the trained staff who are used to giving infusions to children and will know the best methods to calm and comfort them and get them accustomed to the procedure.

Schedule another date night with your spouse.

You don't have to go far, or go for long, or be extravagant, but do go together to some safe place where it is just the two of you for a while. I know you won't be surprised by how much good even a quiet walk around the block, holding hands, will do for you—I'm just reminding you to actually do it.

THE AIR THAT WE BREATHE

HYPERBARICS

AARON

One of my patients' parents once described the atmosphere in my office as "very tightly controlled, very merry chaos." It is a description I love. At any given time, my office is filled with kids playing while they wait to see me; with moms talking together in the waiting room; and with dads stopping by to pick up a refresher supply of nutritional supplements. Other typical visitors will include a doctor who is training with me to learn biomedical protocol; a HEAL! (Healing Every Autistic Life) board member popping in to fill me in on plans for our latest fundraiser; the physical therapist coming over from the office next door to confer about a patient; a football player who needs fixin' after the last game; my nurses giving glutathione infusions and technicians settling children into one of our two hyperbaric chambers for therapy; and my office manager keeping all of us rolling along, more or less on schedule. Meanwhile, this child insists upon finding his favorite nurse and announcing himself immediately upon arrival; that child must have his new toy admired; another child needs me to know that his poops these days are just beautiful before he can settle down to wait his turn; and all of this takes time, not to mention more than a few hugs (and some autographs, too, if one of the football players is around).

Fortunately, I am surrounded by a dedicated and capable staff who flourish in such a fast-paced, nonhierarchical environment—and I have found that my young patients and their parents can relax in the friendliness of an atmosphere that feels very much like a large and loving extended family coordinating their large and exciting lives.

Of course, there are events that ramp even this high-energy outfit up a notch, such as when one of my international patients pays a visit. My waiting room then becomes the base camp for the whole family, every member usually jet lagged and hungry, the kids needing a bottle, a diaper change, a diversion, a nap.

One day in December 2008, Aaron, his parents, and his brother and sister arrived from South Africa. His mom had sought me out several months earlier, when I was in that country training new autism specialists, to ask me to examine her son. Aaron had just been diagnosed with autism, and she was desperate to have him seen by a doctor who wasn't going to consign him, out of hand, to a life of disability. I shuffled around my schedule a little bit and made time to meet Aaron. His mother's determination that I see him notwithstanding, what convinced me to take Aaron on as a patient was the stark fact that if I didn't, he probably wasn't going to get the care he needed. At the time, doctors in his country were just beginning to understand the biomedical model for autism treatment. I couldn't care for every autistic child in South Africa, but I could help this one child. Though I myself often feel as desperate as Aaron's mother in my longing to have the causes of and treatments for autism understood, accepted, and *acted upon* on a global basis, I am also, in many ways, still a typical pediatrician: it is my nature to focus on the individual child right in front of me and to not let him slip through the cracks. The miracle of this approach, though, is that the parents, once their child is on the road to recovery, carry the beacon forward and help to enlighten the rest of the world—often just a few people at a time, but then those few people go out and spread the word to just a few more, and a few more, and a few more, and that's how the whole blessed "payin' it forward" ripple effect starts to work.

Aaron's parents started their whole family on the GFCF diet immediately following our first meeting, and Aaron had progressed rapidly within just weeks of beginning biomedical treatment; within a few years, he'd become one of those children no one would have readily distinguished from a typical kid. Now five years old, he and his whole family were in the United States for one of his follow-up visits. Aaron had made such strides toward recovery that, in fact, I could easily look forward to the day when he would lose his diagnosis. Part of the reason for this joyful prognosis was that we had intervened early in his illness. His parents had suffered from none of the denial that sometimes strikes parents, as it had struck me, when their child is first becoming sick. They knew something was wrong with their beautiful little boy and they had taken him immediately to a doctor who'd diagnosed him and, just as immediately, found a biomedical practitioner—in this case, me—to start him on his healing path.

Another part of the reason for Aaron's remarkably positive response was that his parents were absolutely unwavering in following Aaron's prescribed diet and supplement routine, about killing yeast, and about keeping him on his methyl-B_{12} shot schedule. Now they were ready to commit just as aggressively to the next step of therapy: hyperbarics.

Aaron had, actually, already begun hyperbaric therapy before that visit. He had already completed around 20 hours in a hyperbaric chamber. His progress had so accelerated during the course of his hyperbaric therapy that his parents had decided they needed to make it even more accessible to their son than the overloaded schedule at their local clinic would allow—so they made the investment and purchased a hyperbaric chamber for their home so that Aaron could benefit from open-ended time spent in the chamber.

That day, in my office, in addition to the usual base-camp operations of a weary, traveling family—ordering in lunch, rooting through suitcases to find appropriate clothing for the Florida weather, and stocking up on crates of supplements that might not be readily available in the patient's home country—we were making arrangements for the installation of a hyperbaric chamber in a home half a world away. Meanwhile, Aaron and his mom climbed into one of our hyperbaric chambers together. The hour in the chamber would, for Aaron, help him further along the path of autism recovery and would, for Mom, help her emerge relieved from some of the worst of her jet lag. While Mom and Aaron cuddled up for an hour's nap together, my staff took charge of Aaron's brother and sister so that Dad could concentrate on learning how to use the hyperbaric unit and install it in their house in South Africa.

The confidence Aaron's family has in hyperbaric therapy was earned—they had witnessed Aaron's progress though a series of sessions in a chamber before deciding that it was so valuable they wanted to have it available in their own home. And their confidence is well placed in spite of some uneven media reports about the therapy over the years.

Unfortunately, the only thing most people associate with hyperbarics is the chamber Michael Jackson, the pop singer, reportedly slept in. For some, the singer's erratic behavior and checkered past cast a shadow over his every association—*whacko* became a word they applied not only to him, but to his every undertaking, including hyperbarics.

While hyperbarics has been indiscriminately, and wrongly, touted in the past as a cure-all—and various inappropriate applications have resulted in some deserved backlash from the medical community and in the media—let's not throw out the baby with the bath water. Hyperbaric therapy is, in fact, a credible and highly worthwhile medical therapy.

A BRIEF HISTORY OF HYPERBARIC THERAPY

The word *hyperbaric* means, literally, "high pressure." Hyperbaric oxygen therapy (HBOT) employs oxygen concentrated under high pressure. It is a therapy for injury and disease that was first explored hundreds of years ago.

It was in 1662 that a British clergyman known as Henshaw first used a bellows to control airflow and create increased pressure to "help digestions, to promote insensible respiration, to facilitate breathing, and expectoration and consequently [is] of excellent use for prevention of most affections of the lungs," as is noted in Henshaw's earliest reports on the new discovery. Henshaw's invention to do all of this was called a Domicilium, and it worked by increasing pressure only, without an increase of oxygen concentration—which is understandable given that the element oxygen had yet to be either discovered or named, and wouldn't be for over another hundred years.

In the 1800s, in Europe, and to a lesser degree in America, time in hyperbaric chambers was commonly recommended to patients who suffered from conditions such as asthma, emphysema, chronic bronchitis, and anemia. Not until the 1930s, however, and then only because the United States military had taken an interest in the therapy after World War I, was hyperbarics recognized as a conventional therapy, its credibility bolstered because it had proved successful in treating deep-sea divers suffering from decompression sickness.

Since the 1950s, clinical trials have been ongoing as researchers look to discover other beneficial applications of hyperbaric therapy. But not until the relatively recent use of lower pressure, a phenomenon deeply appreciated by the human brain for its gentler and therefore better tolerated approach to neurologic healing, along with the development of high-tech equipment such as magnetic resonance imaging (MRI) and single photon emission computed tomography (SPECT), has it been possible to investigate and appreciate the beneficial effects of the therapy on neurologic problems. By performing both pre- and posthyperbaric examinations with functional MRI and SPECT technologies, researchers have been able to evaluate and document improvement in a patient's neurologic condition through exposure to hyperbaric oxygen.

These days, there is photographic evidence of, for example, a damaged colon that has been healed or is healing after the patient has undergone hyperbaric therapy. In part because such photographs offer irrefutable evidence of its efficacy, hyperbaric therapy is now increasingly used as part of the treatment for a wide variety of medical conditions. It has been used in as therapy in cases of carbon monoxide poisoning. It has been used to treat brain, nerve, and cardiovascular disorders, as well as the digestive disorders that Henshaw had had a very early inkling would respond to hyperbaric therapy. It has been used to promote the healing of stubbornly non-healing wounds—such as foot wounds resulting from diabetes—and to mitigate damage caused by radiation treatments. It has been used to revitalize blood flow in victims of asphyxiation—near drowning, near hanging, exposure to carbon monoxide, and sleep apnea. It has been used with great success in stroke and multiple sclerosis patients, to heal acute thermal burns, and to promote skin graft acceptance. Hyperbarics, as you see, has many applications, and the role it can play in wellness and preventative care is just beginning to be identified and implemented. And it has, of course, been used to promote healing in autistic kids.

How did hyperbarics become such a big part of autism and recovery? It's appropriate, given my love for the sport, that it should have been through football. In February 2005, Jacksonville hosted the Super Bowl. And a player named Terrell Owens was using a hyperbaric chamber to do the impossible—a season-ending ankle injury that was six weeks old and had been operated upon was going to be healed enough for him to play in the Game. TO hooked up with hyperbarics through a fellow named Bill Schindler. A former Olympic wrestler, Bill had both football players and special needs children using chambers with tremendous success at the Hyperbaric Therapy Center in Atlanta, Georgia. Bill walked into my office while he was here for the Super Bowl and talked to me about *affordable* hyperbarics for autism patients using portable low-pressure chambers. He brought TO's chamber into the office the Monday after the Game, before he headed back to Atlanta, and we gave hyperbarics a whirl with a few children whose parents had read about it and were eager to try it. Those first children showed some pretty impressive changes with just one hour of the therapy, so the families insisted we find a way to bring one into the office, and boy oh boy! did we ever see some neat things start to happen! The rest, as they say, is history!

How does hyperbaric therapy work? How is it that hyperbaric therapy has such a positive impact on patients suffering from such a broad range of injuries and disease?

Hyperbaric therapy is based on what is known in physics as Henry's Law. Formulated by William Henry in 1803, the law states: "At a constant temperature, the amount of a given gas dissolved in a given type and volume of liquid is directly proportional to the partial pressure of that gas in equilibrium with that liquid."

In more everyday language, what that means is that the ability of a gas to dissolve in any liquid is increased when pressure on the liquid is increased. More specifically, as this law applies to hyperbaric therapy, it means that when a patient is exposed to oxygen under pressure (the gas in question), more of the oxygen is dissolved in the patient's blood (the liquid) than it would be at normal atmospheric pressures.

Your next question is bound to be, why is it good to have an increased oxygen supply in your blood? Oxygen, that odorless, colorless gas that makes up little more than 20 percent of our atmosphere, is essential to life. On a very practical level, we're all aware of just how urgent it is to have enough air to breathe. Of the elemental conditions necessary to sustain life, a human being can do without water to drink, depending on weather conditions and exertion levels, for up to three to ten days, and without food to eat for several weeks. Survival has even been accomplished by people who have gone without food for several months. But the amount of time that we can do without oxygen is measured in minutes.

However basic oxygen is to us on a minute-by-minute basis, most of us take air for granted. We don't realize that oxygen is a major ingredient of every component of our body—water, protein, fat—or that it is critical not just as the gas with which we happen to fill our lungs, but also as the agent that metabolizes glucose in our bodies, producing the energy the body needs to perform functions such as respiration, circulation, and digestion and helping it to maintain a constant body temperature. When we don't get *any* oxygen, our bodies die; when we don't get *enough* oxygen, the body ceases to function well, and its systems start to shut down. Our breath grows short, our pulse rate increases, our blood pressure drops, our skin and mucous membranes begin to turn blue, our mental capacity is compromised, and we begin to hallucinate—all these are precursor signs that the systems and organs in our body are beginning to shut down for want of air. The name for the impact of a reduced oxygen supply is *hypoxia*—the *under oxygenation* of living tissue. Ultimately, if the oxygen supply is not restored in an extremely timely manner, the result is death.

Normally, oxygen enters our bodies through the act of breathing and is transported through our bodies by our blood. Blood consists of three main components: white blood cells (WBCs) that fight infection; red blood cells (RBCs) that, because of their hemoglobin, do the actual carrying around of the oxygen to all the other places in the body where it is needed; and plasma, the yellowish fluid in which the WBCs and RBCs are suspended, thus enabling them to move through our arteries and veins and capillaries. Our blood, of course, has a variety of other things it carries throughout our bodies as well. It distributes other building blocks of healthy cells, such as proteins, minerals, and hormones. It is the main way that certain waste products of our metabolism, such as carbon dioxide, are excreted. But it is the blood's function of moving oxygen, and the healing aspects of the available supply of oxygen, around which hyperbaric therapy is concentrated.

How does oxygen heal—and how does an increased and pressurized supply of it speed the healing? First things first: it is simply intuitive that, if oxygen is a major component of healthy cell composition and function, a steady supply of it is necessary for the cells to carry out their usual functions of *growing* healthy tissue, muscle, and bone; *defending* against infection; and *repairing* inflammation and other physical damage sustained by the body. These tasks are all carried out at a cellular level. A gently increased supply of oxygen, therefore, nurtures growth, strengthens defense, and promotes speedy repair.

For an analogy, let's look to those poor goldfish so many kids win as prizes at street fairs. The prize fish was likely delivered to the winner in a sealed plastic baggie. Often, even before the winner can arrive back at his house, the little fish is dead. That's because it has used up all the oxygen available in the sealed baggie and has suffocated—a cruel end for the innocent fish. If the fish survives his move, and is placed in one of those classic, wide-mouthed glass fishbowls filled with clean water as soon as it is possible, the amount of oxygen that is in the water, as well as the amount that is able to enter the fishbowl through the wide mouth, will allow the fish to sustain life for several days, or maybe weeks. The wider the mouth of the fishbowl—that is, the larger the surface of the water—the more oxygen that can enter the water and the longer the fish will live.

If, however, the fish's new home is an aquarium fitted with an oxygen pump that supplies a constant stream of fresh oxygen directly into the water, the fish will likely have a long and happy life.

Think of a hyperbaric chamber as an oxygen aquarium, an environment where a supply of fresh oxygen is pumped in a constant stream.

In a hyperbaric chamber, however, the supply of oxygen is more than just constant. It is also pressurized. This allows for the oxygen level in the body to be increased many times greater than normal. Outside of the sealed, pressurized chamber, it is impossible, no matter how deeply or yogic-ly one breathes, for a person to come close to increasing her oxygen levels to this extent.

How does the pressure of a hyperbaric chamber raise a person's oxygen level? Under normal atmospheric conditions, almost 98 percent of the body's oxygen supply is carried around the bloodstream bound to hemoglobin, bound to the RBCs, and the remaining approximately 2 percent is dissolved in the plasma. Under hyperbaric pressure, oxygen dissolves directly into the plasma. When that oxygen arrives at its destination, it behaves differently than oxygen that is bound to hemoglobin. Oxygen bound to hemoglobin travels a fixed distance into tissues. Oxygen dissolved in plasma behaves according to diffusion laws, and the diffusion gradient allows oxygen dissolved in plasma to wash up onto the shore of human tissues like a tsunami wave.

The oxygen is carried, for instance, to the upper-arm hematoma that one of my football players sustained after a nasty tackle. In this case, the extra oxygen helps his body reduce the inflammation associated with the hematoma and also helps the body to break up and remove the clotted blood—the bruise—that was the physical evidence of the trauma the tissue sustained.

For a stroke victim, the extra oxygen making its way to the damaged areas of the brain where the stroke occurred awakens the many dormant, but not dead, cells surrounding the affected area. With this awakening of the cells in the area known as the *ischemic penumbra* comes, often, significant improvement for folks with "old" strokes whose status is presumed to be fixed, stagnant, and static.

The positive effects of hyperbaric therapy for autistic kids are just as dramatic—we see jaw-dropping changes from pre- to post-therapy brain SPECT scans of our children that correlate with restoring function to a dormant area of a brain. As hyperbarics works for stroke patients—resulting in restored speech and muscle control—so it works for autism patients. But the results can seem even more pronounced in autistic kids. That is because in autism, so many areas of the body—so many systems—become dysfunctional, and hyperbarics addresses all of them, simultaneously. A leaky gut? The extra oxygen helps to repair the very "holes" in the intestinal tissue. A distressed immune system? The extra oxygen increases the ability of WBCs to fight infection. The photographic evidence of irritable colons before and after hyperbaric therapy is particularly striking: where once the colon was swollen, discolored, and filled with "pockets," the posttreatment colon is smooth and pink.

HYPERBARICS FOR EVERYONE

I am a proponent of the benefits of hyperbaric therapy in wellness. The physiological effects of the therapy may be more apparent for those who are suffering from a diagnosed illness, but they can also be a significant part of preventative medical care. Let me break down some of these benefits:

- A low level of oxygen reduces the body's ability to fight off invading bacteria, but the reoxygenation of the tissue has an apparently antibacterial effect.
- Hyperbaric therapy has been shown to increase the body's ability to make new bone cells, healing fractures more quickly and slowing progression of osteoporosis.
- Toxins lodged in the body—*everybody's* body, though not as densely as the volume autistic kids carry around—are likely broken down and flushed away by the additional oxygen, though proving this will require more research.

- Extra oxygen, provided at low pressures in modest amounts, in the brain area allows for sharpened mental acuity—or, improved *cerebral metabolism,* the rate at which the brain can work—critical for autistic children, and helpful to all of us, especially seniors who may be starting to be forgetful.
- Oxygen is a powerful anti-inflammatory agent, relieving joint pain and restoring mobility and range of motion.

These benefits I've just listed don't encompass the limits of what hyperbaric therapy may—in conjunction with other treatments, from increased dietary nutrition to, in some cases, surgery—be able to accomplish. I'm confident there are many other, yet-undiscovered ways in which this therapy can be helpful. For example, because hyperbaric treatment increases oxygen levels in spinal fluid, it is now being used to treat spinal injuries and paralysis with some success. Once again, football has been responsible for instructing me in these possibilities. In early 2008, I was asked to help J. T. Townsend. When I met him, this charming young man was a twenty-one-year old quadriplegic whose certain future playing in the NBA or NFL had abruptly ended four years before, when he sustained a C1 spinal sprain on the football field in his senior year in high school. The day he rolled into my office with just a little movement in his arms and neck to try out hyperbarics, I wondered how much improvement we'd get. It wasn't long before therapists were watching muscles fire in his legs and feet. Using aggressive hyperbarics and now adding intense rehabilitative physical therapy, we are in dogged pursuit of strength and function. As with most of my patients, J. T. is now part of our extended family—we all take a personal stake in each other's progress; my daughter watches J. T.'s progress and has told us her goal is to dance with him some day.

Still, hyperbaric therapy is not, as I said when we first started talking about it, a cure-all. In fact there are some contraindications and cautions for the therapy—it should not be administered to people suffering from acute ear or sinus infections, for example, and, possibly, to pregnant women.

It is, however, a therapy that, through boosting the supply of an element the body relies on naturally to grow, defend, and repair itself, can both greatly enhance the effectiveness of other therapeutic treatments as well as preserve and protect the integrity of already-healthy cells.

WHEN, AND HOW MUCH?

Just about every autistic child for whom I have recommended HBOT has benefited from the therapy. Indeed, the more profoundly impacted the child is by the disease, the more obvious the benefits appear to be. Conversely, the more subtle the abnormalities of the child, the more subtle the improvement, though even children with diagnoses of ADD and some learning disabilities often improve with this therapy.

When to start hyperbaric therapy for an autism patient is very much a matter of the personal preference of the physician. In my practice, I like to stabilize the child's diet and nutrient supplementation and look closely at the individual patient's sulfation and methylation issues and begin to support these two areas first. This gives us a baseline to refer to when we begin hyperbarics. The results we have achieved in this way are tremendous, with our children making strides in several key, observable areas:

- speech, language, and communication
- sociability and "presence" in our world
- cognitive and sensory awareness
- focus and concentration
- sleep patterns
- bowel function
- general behavior, including cooperation (for example, in school, probably because it is so much easier to learn when you feel good!).

The neurological benefits usually start to become apparent after about ten hours of the therapy, and the results I have seen in my patients appear to be not only sustained, but to grow even after the therapy is discontinued. There doesn't seem to be an end point to how much they will grow, either; with hyperbaric therapy there is no known point where improvement ceases. My recommendation is that parents start their kids with a commitment to spend 40 hours in a hyperbaric chamber, in increments of 60- to 90-minute sessions over the course of several months. After 40 hours of therapy, the great majority of kids show some amazing gains in cognition as well as in other areas. Older or more profoundly impacted children may need more time before they show the signs of the benefits they are receiving. Why 40 hours? Forty hours has been the convention of most research, and so has become the tradition in thinking about hyperbarics and durations of therapy.

When the first 40 hours of sessions are completed, if feasible, I recommend that my patients continue the therapy in intermittent 40-hour "pulses," always keeping a record of the gains each unique child makes along the way. The pulses can be important in allowing us to track improvement. Additionally, hyperbaric therapy also seems to positively impact vision. While this is seemingly a good thing, when it occurs it often takes time for patients to accommodate and adjust to increased clarity of eyesight. If it is feasible for families who see excellent results, I am happy for them to continue hyperbaric therapy as part of long-term wellness maintenance, taking advantage of the overall health benefits we've touched on in this chapter.

Often, however, I don't have to even recommend this: a parent, or another adult of the parents' choosing, is required to accompany younger children into the chamber for their sessions. We do this simply so that the child will have company and remain comfortable throughout the session, and so that they will not attempt an early exit from a pressurized chamber. But because of this rule, Mom and/or Dad are also experiencing the healing aspects of the therapy personally. While they can't always tell me what exactly feels better, Mom and Dad often feel better too. A knee, in the past stiff due to an old injury, no longer gives them trouble on rainy days, or they are sleeping more deeply and waking more rested, or they find they are just able to concentrate better at work and be more efficient at their job. Often, after parents have experienced the real physical glow you feel after a hyperbaric session, they simply ask to stay on the therapy after they complete their first 40 hours.

What is a typical hyperbaric session like?

A hyperbaric session is quite a simple procedure for the patient in our low pressure, less than 100 percent oxygen chambers. Shoes come off. But other than that, patients wear their street clothes into the chamber. We, of course, recommend that adults accompanying the patient stop use of tobacco products altogether as they significantly interfere with the body's ability to transport oxygen. The only other constraint is not using perfume or aftershave; scents are tremendously intensified under pressure and can make anyone feel ill while in a hyperbaric chamber.

The chamber itself looks like a large, collapsed plastic cylinder from the outside. Inside, once inflated, it is more spacious than most folks anticipate—about the same amount of room as in the lower bunk of a set of bunk beds—but, in my office, filled with blankets and pillows and, if the child decides upon it, a stuffed animal or two, so that the space for two people often gets cozy. The wondrous part of this fact is that while in the chamber, our children seem to feel more affectionate and snuggly than they have in months or years, something most mommies and daddies treasure.

The patient is then zipped into the chamber, and a technician starts to inflate the unit. While the chamber is inflating and coming up to pressure, the patient may begin to feel just like he does on a plane during takeoff and landing—that is, his ear and sinus pressure may take a few minutes to equalize. The same tricks you'd use in an actual airplane to fix that problem apply: swallowing, yawning, or gently trying to blow through your nose while you are holding it. And of course, our technicians carefully control the rate of pressurization, ensuring that there is no discomfort for the patient.

When the unit is fully pressurized, the patient gets comfortable—there is a technician outside who is closely monitoring the session. The patient can even see and talk to the technician through a clear plastic window located by her head. Inside, the patient can read, listen to an iPod, watch one of the DVDs he's chosen from our extensive stash of kid favorites, or simply take a nap.

The average session lasts from 60 to 90 minutes, though the only real limit on the amount of time you can spend in the unit is dictated by the fact that hyperbaric therapy makes you want to pee. Younger kids sometimes wear diapers for their sessions, and more than one mom has made a beeline for the rest room at the end of the session. It may surprise you, then, to know that many of my patients appreciate the benefits of hyperbaric therapy so much that, like Aaron's family, they have a unit in their homes and often spend more than an hour each day in them. Actually, Dani and I often have our best Mommy/Dani time in the chamber. Hyperbaric therapy both promotes healing and preserves health. Our hours in the chamber foster Dani's continued recovery, give us much needed snuggle time, and are part of a healthy lifestyle that allows me to keep up with her.

VISIT #4

ACTION LIST

Review your child's diet and nutritional supplement program with your practitioner and make any adjustments that are necessary or seem prudent.

This review of the records you are keeping as a parent can coincide with a review of the child's allergy profile, which your practitioner may or may not have recommended, depending on the child's response to the standard changes required by the GFCF diet. An allergy profile can be an important piece of information to have during the healing process, allowing you to zero in on very specific foods to which your child may be sensitive and remove them from his diet.

Notice and record signs of physical and behavioral improvements.

How is his stimming? Reduced, but not yet completely gone? Does he recognize Grandma when she comes to visit, and does he run to greet her with enthusiasm? Is he completely potty trained yet, if that was an issue? Is he gaining weight? Is his tummy flat? How is her muscle tone? Is her language more spontaneous? Is he still demonstrating obsessive behaviors, and, if so, what seems to be the trigger for them? Discuss the steps your child may have taken—both steps ahead and steps back—so that you and your clinician can make determinations about any changes that seem warranted in, for example, the child's dosage of methyl-B_{12}, or antifungal medications.

Discuss with your doctor any conditions you may have that may preclude hyperbaric treatment.
When your child—and you—are cleared to start hyperbaric therapy, schedule your first series of appointments.

Remember how important family nights and date nights are to your child's recovery and schedule them frequently.

CAN WE CHELATE HIM NOW?

"Can we chelate him *now?*" That's the burning question most parents have either asked me, or have wanted to ask me, from their first appointment. They ask me this earnestly—and desperately. Sometimes, they even ask it furtively, as if they aren't quite sure they're not out of bounds to want to know. They've read all about chelation—its benefits as well as the controversies surrounding it; they're longing to make it part of their child's routine because they want their child back whole—and yet, sometimes, they're afraid of it.

What parents invariably mean when they ask me about chelation is, When can we begin using DMSA (dimercaptosuccinic acid) or EDTA (ethylenediamine tetraacetic acid), one of the FDA-approved medicines to treat heavy metal poisoning? In order for me to answer this question, we need to come to a full understanding of what chelation is and why and when the DMSAs or EDTAs are of value in treating autism.

Chelation is the process of introducing an agent into the body that will attach itself molecularly to a heavy metal, usher it out of the tissue where it is lodged, and flush it into the bloodstream and out of the body by way of the kidneys and liver. This is all chelation really is: introducing an agent into the body to remove heavy metals because the body's own natural detoxification system has gone awry, or because the system is too overloaded with environmental toxins to keep up with the amount of detoxification it is being asked to handle.

Now, think about that. Think about the material we covered in Visit #3: our bodies were designed to produce glutathione, the Yoda of antioxidants—and glutathione has the unique ability to surround particles of heavy metals, squeeze those particles onto itself, lead them to the bloodstream, and flush them out of the body by way of the liver and kidneys.

Gee. That sounds an awful lot like what chelating agents do.

Exactly.

It's likely that by this point in your treatment process, your child has been receiving regular glutathione infusions and/or support of the methylation and sulfation process that synthesizes glutathione for several months. At the very least, support of methylation and sulfation are improving glutathione synthesis. The glutathione is already doing the work of detoxifying her body of the heavy metals. You are already chelating her.

My dear friend Dr. Boyd Haley, of previously mentioned brilliance and acerbic, sarcastic wit, has spent much of his career researching diseases caused, at least in part, by biochemical problems at the molecular level. From Gulf War syndrome to Alzheimer's and ASDs, the discoveries Boyd is making are revolutionizing the quality of care we can offer to our veterans, our elderly, and our autistic kids. As Boyd says, it is completely possible, with time and enough treatments, to chelate using only glutathione and vitamin C. You may be surprised to learn that vitamin C, with which you have likely already been supplementing your child's diet as part of the biomedical protocol, is another natural chelating agent, specifically working to rid the body of aluminum accumulated in brain cells.

So, in understanding chelation, the first thing we have to do is to make a distinction between detoxifying using chelating agents such as glutathione and vitamin C and detoxifying using chelating agents such as DMSA or EDTA. If your child is receiving glutathione infusions, you are already chelating him. So if and when you and your doctor decide to take the next step in the detoxification journey and begin what I'll call "standard chelation therapy"—that is, chelation therapy with a synthetic chelating agent—you are not moving into brand new territory; you are only enhancing a process you have already begun with glutathione and vitamin C.

A BRIEF HISTORY OF CHELATION

Now, for the rest of this chapter, when I talk about chelation, unless I specify otherwise, what I am going to be referring to is "standard chelation therapy"—and that's a therapy that raises some eyebrows in the established medical world, though it's been a standard medical practice for nearly a hundred years.

Doctors first developed and began using chelating agents to treat soldiers who had been exposed to the poisonous gas Lewisite in World War I. Lewisite is an arsenic-based poison gas, and the chelating agent used to treat it was an organic dithiol compound called dimercaprol. It was given the common name British Anti-Lewisite and is usually referred to by its shortened form, BAL. The sulfur atoms in BAL bonded tightly to the arsenic and formed a water-soluble compound that allowed the heavy metal to enter the sufferer's bloodstream and be flushed from his body. That's essentially the same way chelating agents work today, but while BAL did remove the arsenic from the soldiers' bodies, it had some fairly unpleasant—even severe—side effects, such as limiting the air capacity of the lungs.

By World War II, when chelating once again became necessary to the military, advances had been made in the sorts of chemicals used to make chelating agents. Navy personnel began to suffer in large numbers from lead poisoning, the result of being exposed to lead-based paint while painting the hulls of ships. The new chelating agent EDTA was introduced to address the problem. Because, unlike BAL, EDTA was made with a synthetic amino acid, its side effects were less severe.

In the 1960s, the chelating agent DMSA was introduced. It was made by essentially modifying the BAL formula using a different dithiol that tempered BAL's noted side effects. Since that time, chelation with DMSA has become one of the standard forms of care for the treatment of heavy metal poisoning—poisoning caused by arsenic, lead, and mercury.

Public understanding of chelation therapy—and the incredible good that it had the potential to do—hit a zenith in 1976 when Harold McCluskey, a chemical operations technician at the Hanford Plutonium Finishing Plant in Washington state, was poisoned with the highest dose of americium radiation ever recorded. Mr. McCluskey became known in the press as the "Atomic Man" when an accident at the plant caused an explosion that exposed him to 500 times the occupational standard for americium 241, a plutonium by-product.

For five months, Mr. McCluskey lived in isolation at the Hanford Emergency Decontamination Facility—because there was a risk that in interacting with other people he would contaminate them too—and he underwent chelation therapy using the chelating agent DTPA. Within a year, his radiation count had fallen by approximately 80 percent and his doctors deemed him ready to emerge from isolation. Though it took his minister stepping forward to convince others that it was once again safe for them to be around Mr. McCluskey, he lived for 11 more years and died at the age of 75 from coronary artery disease.

How did a process like chelation evolve from a standard, safe, medically approved therapy that famously saved the life of "Atomic Man" to one that is today desperately—even furtively—sought out by parents of autistic kids?

MERCURY POISONING AND AUTISM

Part of the reason that chelation therapy has become controversial is that it may have been used in some questionable applications. There is a theory, for example, that chelation therapy can be helpful in the treatment of atherosclerosis, or hardening of the arteries, by helping to remove deposits of fat, cholesterol, and calcium from the artery walls. Whether this is a valid application or not I do not know—and unfortunately, the trials that might have enlightened all of us were scrapped in September 2008 after an extensive lobbying effort. This effort included such agencies as the National Heart, Lung, and Blood Institute of the National Institutes of Health (NIH) weighing in against conducting the clinical study of chelation and atherosclerosis with an oxymoronic logic that, in essence, went something like this: not enough clinical studies had yet been done to prove that this clinical study was needed.

The larger reason chelation is controversial, specifically to the treatment of autism, is that chelation is a therapy classically used to treat heavy metal poisoning, and the medical establishment has not yet admitted that autism is, in fact, a toxic condition. It has not yet faced up to the fact that autism *is* a manifestation of heavy metal poisoning, both direct and indirect, though even a cursory look at the similarities between the two conditions makes it obvious to even a disinterested layperson. Let's compare the signs and symptoms of autism and mercury poisoning right here (just as did Sally Bernard, who was the lead author on the originally published comparison), so that you can make up your own mind about it.

The psychiatric disturbances associated with mercury poisoning are social deficits, shyness, social withdrawal, depression, mood swings, mask face, schizoid tendencies, OCD traits, lack of eye contact, irrational fears, irritability, aggression, temper tantrums, and impaired face recognition. The psychiatric disturbances for autism? Social deficits, shyness, social withdrawal, depressive traits, mood swings, flat affect, schizoid tendencies, OCD traits, lack of eye contact, irrational fears, irritability, aggression, temper tantrums, and impaired face recognition.

The speech, language, and hearing deficits associated with mercury poisoning are loss of speech or failure to develop speech, articulation problems, sound sensitivity, hearing loss—or, in the case of high doses of mercury, deafness—and poor performance on language IQ tests. For autism? Delayed speech or failure to develop speech, articulation problems, sound sensitivity, mild to profound hearing loss, and poor performance on language IQ tests.

Sensory abnormalities that result from mercury poisoning include involuntary jerking movements such as arm flapping, ankle jerking, circling, and rocking. For autism, the stereotypical movements include arm flapping, ankle jerking, circling, and rocking. Cognitive impairments? Sufferers of both conditions share the same assumptions of borderline intelligence and mental retardation, which is "reversible" in the case of mercury poisoning and "sometimes recoverable" in autism. Regarding unusual behaviors, sufferers share the same tendencies to experience ADHD traits, sleep difficulties, eating disorders and feeding problems, and self-injurious behaviors such as head banging.

Even more tellingly, both conditions share the exact same physical and biochemical disturbances. Even the briefest and most noninclusive list of these shared problems is striking: incontinence, skin rashes, elevated heart rate, diarrhea, constipation, abdominal pain, leaky gut syndrome, low sulfate and glutathione levels, allergies and food sensitivities, asthma, decreased serotonin levels, demyelization of the brain, and seizures.

In September of 2008, the National Institute of Mental Health (NIMH) called off its proposed study of chelation therapy for autism that could have once and for all removed any doubt that lingers in the minds of skeptics about chelation as appropriate and enormously effective in this application. The study, stalled over actual research design, had been in the planning stages for two years, so when the NIMH abandoned it, you can imagine the intense disappointment and anger that was experienced in the autism community. If performed in the manner in which those of us who regularly use chelation do it, the study would likely have proven the efficacy of chelation for autism. This would have unquestionably established the link between autism and mercury poisoning—and that link would have opened up the whole can of worms I have decided I'm not going to open in this book.

However, the fact remains that in practice, careful chelation can be as effective for autistic patients as it is for those suffering from mercury poisoning. Those of us in the biomedical field fully understand that autism and mercury poisoning are joined at the hip. Autism looks like mercury poisoning. It quacks like mercury poisoning. It waddles like mercury poisoning. So we call it what it is, mercury poisoning, and we treat it like that too, with chelation. And chelation—whether with glutathione, vitamin C, or another chelating agent—is what has brought us the great success in recovery that we have enjoyed. All we have to do is be willing to call a duck a goddamned duck.

STARTING CHELATION

All right, now we know that chelation is a safe, standard medical procedure for helping the body to get rid of the heavy metals that make it sick—and we also know that autism is a most correct application of the therapy. When is the right time to begin to chelate?

When I was a resident, I did a surgical rotation and even considered making surgery my specialty. In order to perform surgery efficiently and safely, there are any number of dominoes you've got to align: the operating room needs to be properly staffed, the anesthesia must be administered, and the patient must be appropriately prepped and draped before you begin whatever procedure you are undertaking. Even then, a surgeon doesn't just plunge into a patient with the scalpel; she begins with the outermost layer and proceeds in an orderly fashion through each layer of skin and muscle tissue to get to wherever the trouble is.

When you want to sew a dress, you start out not by cutting the fabric but by cutting out and ironing the pattern pieces, then washing and pressing the fabric before pinning the pattern pieces to it, and only then do you pick up a scissors to cut material. In the kitchen, if you are just beginning to cook, you learn to make toast and boil an egg before you attempt to pick up Emeril Lagasse's most complicated recipe and replicate it.

You get the idea: you don't begin to chelate until you have successfully completed all the other steps I've outlined through the course of this book—weaning your child from gluten and casein, strengthening her system with a good supplement program, killing yeast, and starting to normalize her compromised sulfate metabolism and methylation chemistries. To begin chelation, your child's body must be stabilized in all these ways, and that is because chelation can be physically stressful. Her body has got to be fortified to tolerate this stress. Remember that we got into this mess in the first place because this particular body had trouble managing and excreting metals. It is wise to support and repair those compromised processes before asking them to work overtime. It is also more than wise, it is critical, to have a physician monitoring this medical procedure.

The benefits of chelation are many, and its goal is a more sustainable recovery from autism so that the child is physically and mentally able to resume the typical life he was meant to lead prior to getting sick. It is the process of detoxification that should allow the gut to heal, the immune system to function more normally, and so on. Before beginning, we need to address the possible side effects to chelation; what you don't want are the side effects impinging on the child's overall health and well-being—the cure, so to speak, being worse than the disease. The side effects can include a burning sensation at the site where the chelating agent is delivered into the vein, which is controllable, as well as the more rare reactions such as headache, nausea, stomach upset, vomiting, and fever. In some children, the chelating agent can yield symptoms that may be yeast overgrowth or may be inadequate sulfation support masquerading as yeast overgrowth. This is yet another reason for ensuring good sulfation support and for controlling and maintaining control of any yeast infestation before beginning the therapy.

Perhaps one of chelation's most notorious side effects is that of acute hypocalcemia, an initially asymptomatic drop in calcium in the bloodstream that can quickly become a serious problem. But here's the part people fail to mention when cautioning parents about chelation—there is only one medication that is guilty of causing this problem. Avoid sodium EDTA and instead use calcium EDTA, and the problem simply does not occur.

Knowing about these possible side effects is the first step in preventing them. It is my firm conviction that children simply should not have to feel poorly while they are excreting the metals that are making them sick. In my years of practice, I have not had issues with the side effects during chelation, and that is because, when it comes to this stage of the recovery process, I am even more extremely cautious than I usually am. I begin with infinitesimal doses of the chelating agent and only very slowly, over the course of weeks and months, depending on the response of the individual child, increase the amount. You remember that old story of the tortoise and the hare? When it comes to chelation, I am a tortoise. Recovery from autism is not a race for the showy and speedy—as I've been repeating all along, it is a marathon for the slow and steady, for those with the patience and faith to pace themselves to win.

CHELATING AGENTS

There are many different chelating agents for your clinician to choose among when deciding on the right prescription for your child. Some of the more common names you'll hear include DMSA, dimercapto-propsane sulfonate (DMPS), and EDTA. The names may seem confusing, but there are some very clear-cut ways in which your clinician will decide which one to use. His decision will be based on several factors: particular characteristics of your child's biochemistry that can indicate the suitability of one type of agent over another; your child's general health and stability to this point in the biomedical process; and the doctor's preference based on results he has previously achieved using each type of agent.

One determining factor will be the fact that different chelating agents have affinities for different metals. For example, in order for an agent to be a good chelator of mercury, its molecules must have a structure that allows it to bind well to mercury—that's two opposed sulfhydryl groups, for the chemically inclined. These two opposed groups allow the chelating molecule to "pinch" hold of the mercury molecule and make it very hard for the mercury molecule to get away. On the other hand, compounds that have only one sulfhydryl group are not as effective as chelators because they don't pinch the metal tightly enough and it's easy for the metal to get away and bind to another molecule—and that means the metal may not be flushed *out* of the body, but only moved to another place *in* the body. DMSA, though designed for chelation of lead, is a good mercury chelator; it's not terribly picky about what metal it bonds to, but once it gets hold, it hangs on like a terrier and doesn't let go.

TRACKING MERCURY

Blood tests show that in comparison to typical children, autistic kids have what are plainly horrifying levels of a variety of chemicals in their small and vulnerable systems. I won't talk about the various units of measure here, for that is not what is striking. What is horrifying is the *magnitude* of differences, the *manifold* differences in the quantities found in typical children and in children with autism.

Aroclors, which are commercial mixtures of PCB compounds (any family of industrial compounds produced by the chlorination of biphenyl), regularly found in common household products such as caulking, wood floor finishes, paints, and antidust agents, show up in a range of 1 to 4 in typical kids, and 50 to 84 in those with autism. Benzene, a known carcinogen and natural constituent of crude oil, shows up in a range of 65 to 140 for typical kids and 240 to 540 in our autistic kids. Dry-cleaning fluid shows up in typical kids in a range of 30 to 110, but for autistic kids it skyrockets up to 688 at the high end. The amount of these environmental toxins in our kids' systems is measurable.

Mercury is not nearly as measurable.

If you've ever played with a ball of pure mercury, tried rolling it around between your fingers—which, astonishingly, was something science teachers frequently allowed their students to do not so very long ago—you know how slippery it is. You'll know why it is sometimes called quicksilver and just how accurate it is to describe a short-tempered friend as "mercurial."

Similarly, mercury is slippery when it's inside the body. It is very hard to find evidence of mercury in the human body—in blood or urine or hair. In just a few short months after mercury exposure ends, there will be no detectible trace of the element in the conventional tests for heavy metals. That's because organs that are not part of the body's central nervous system gradually rid themselves of mercury, but the mercury that stays behind is tightly bound within the liver, kidney, the lining of the GI tract, and the brain. This is why many children, especially older children, who have been diagnosed with autism will show no signs of mercury poisoning after conventional testing—the mercury is settled too deeply into their systems, and none of it is any longer leeching out. The mercury has settled in, indeed, for the long haul. In the brain, mercury has a half-life of about 20 years—a far longer time than in any other organ outside of the central nervous system. At this point, within just those few short months after the exposure ends, the only way to test for it with reliability is to do a biopsy—obviously, not a recommended procedure.

So, then, how will you know when the chelation is working? Well, the obvious answer, from a clinician's standpoint, is that you will see your child's gradual and sustained improvement. Unfortunately, this method of measuring whether chelation is working is not sufficient for those who require more precise measures of success, such as courts and insurance companies. And thus we find ourselves trying to quantify excretion of toxins with laboratory tests.

Periodically during chelation treatment, your practitioner will run several tests. These tests—urine and stool and blood tests—will attempt to monitor and quantify the excretion of metals through the effect of chelation on your child's body. The urine and stool tests may also help you and your doctor determine the length of time the chelation process needs to last: because each child's biochemical system is unique, and because each child's level of exposure will have been to some degree different, there is no precise way to predict when you will be able to end the therapy. Chelation therapy continues until no more metals appear in the periodic urine and stool test results, but more importantly, until no further clinical gains are being made with it. Typically, this period lasts from several months to several years.

Oh, and one other test that is commonly used to check for mercury poisoning in the event the exposure is not recent and therefore may not show up in conventional blood tests? Doctors check for low plasma sulfate levels. Low plasma sulfate levels can be an indication of mercury poisoning.

Yes, you read that right.

It's well documented in the medical literature that 73 to 92 percent of autistic kids have low plasma sulfate levels. The fact that low plasma sulfate levels are themselves used as evidence of mercury poisoning is just one more indication that, indeed, it's really a duck we're dealing with here.

HOW TO PREPARE FOR CHELATION

In addition to having your doctor determine that your child is suitably stable enough to begin chelation, there are several things you'll need to do to prepare for the therapy.

The first thing to do, if you haven't already done it, is to make sure all fish and seafood are removed from your child's diet. Fish and seafood are real, potential sources of the very metal you're trying to remove from the child's system. My daughter, Dani, is one of those possibly rare kids who really likes fish. Though we never serve it at home, she likes it so much that she tries to order it for dinner whenever we go out to a restaurant to eat. I admit that sometimes I let her, as long as it's a fish known to be low in mercury and I know her glutathione support is in good order. But as you're going through chelation therapy, you'll need to be strict about the no fish/no seafood rule.

Next, your doctor will want to take several tests to establish a baseline for your child's blood count, kidney and liver functions, and mineral levels. Mineral levels are especially important to monitor through the chelation process as the traditional chelating agents can sometimes bond with these essential nutrients and flush them out along with the heavy metals. These tests will be part of the series of tests your doctor will order every two or three months (along with the urine and stool tests that check for metal excretion); you'll be able to track your child's mineral levels in this way and adjust her supplement schedule to increase her mineral intake if necessary.

Finally, because there are potential side effects with chelation that could become serious if not monitored, the only way that it is safe to chelate is in a medical setting, under medical supervision. I'm telling you this because over-the-counter chelating methods do exist, and I don't recommend them. They are especially inappropriate for autistic kids for two reasons. First and foremost, a doctor's supervision of chelation is imperative to ensure that your child's delicate systems are monitored sufficiently during the chelation process, and this can only happen with regular visits with your physician and needed laboratory testing. Second, not all chelating methods are efficient or reliable, and many are not a good use of family funds.

There are several ways to chelate reliably, and transdermally *is* one of them, but with prescription topical lotions. There are oral chelation methods as well as suppositories. In my experience, though most of these methods work reasonably well, IV chelation produces the most effective results. An infusion normally takes between 30 minutes and 1 hour to perform. Again, though your child will have to be prepared to deal with yet another needle in his life, he will likely begin to feel so much better as a result of the therapy that the new needle will come to seem like a minor inconvenience in comparison.

CHELATION BOOSTERS

In addition to chelation itself, there are several avenues you will want to explore to boost the efficacy of the therapy, or to mitigate some of the more minor side effects. Your doctor will likely have his or her own recommendations culled from long experience with the chelation process. Here are a few of mine.

N-acetylcysteine.

N-acetylcysteine (NAC) is a pharmaceutical used mainly as a mucolytic agent—an expectorant. We use it in our infusions, though, because of the cysteine part of this molecule. Cysteine is the immediate precursor to glutathione in the glutathione synthesis process. So NAC is a building block that helps the child to make more glutathione over the short term.

Activated Charcoal.

Activated charcoal is a form of carbon that has been processed so that it is extremely porous and, therefore, has a very large surface area. In its oral form, it is routinely administered by emergency response technicians in cases of suspected poisonings or overdoses as it will bind to any toxins in the system and absorb them into its large, porous surface, thus preventing the toxins from being absorbed by the GI tract. If the child is demonstrating any symptoms that the detoxification process is irritating her body, giving her activated charcoal can ameliorate the symptoms, allowing her body a respite from all its hard work.

Far Infrared Sauna Therapy.

To understand how this therapy can be a good adjunct to chelation, it's necessary to have just a small understanding of how infrared (IR) energy works. IR radiation is not at all the same as ultraviolet (UV) radiation that causes sunburn, or atomic (nuclear) radiation. Indeed, almost 80 percent of the sun's rays are IR, and they are not only harmless to us, but it is with the help of these rays that we make indispensable vitamin D in our bodies.

IR consists of radiant heat waves invisible to the human eye; its wave lengths are measured in microns (μm), which are one-one-millionth of a meter. Our atmosphere allows IR rays of 7 to 14 μm (middle to far IR range in the electromagnetic spectrum) to safely reach the earth's surface. The healthy human body, as it happens, also radiates IR energy through the skin in the average range of about 9 μm. Far IR Sauna therapy duplicates the healthy frequencies of our cells, apparently allowing sick cells to normalize and boosting the healing process of cells in crisis.

As you will note from reading about these adjunct therapies, the key concept of *balance* applies to every part of biomedical intervention, including chelation. Is the child's system balanced enough to enhance the chelating effects of glutathione and vitamin C with a more aggressive chelating agent? Is the child detoxing too rapidly? Then let's slow down the process with activated charcoal or altered doses of our infusion components. Is the child showing brilliant progress in the new phase of chelation? Then let's see if we can tweak it up a notch with a little more calcium EDTA or glutathione. Is the child feeling run down, or behaving lethargically? Well, what can we do to help? Adjust his nutrient supplements? Check to see if there is a yeast recurrence we need to be addressing? Increase the frequency of his hyperbaric sessions? Would Far IR Sauna therapy speed his healing—should we start a schedule of that therapy and monitor the results? Should we back off from chelation for a few weeks until he regains his balance?

As I said earlier in this book, biomedical intervention is not a silver bullet. A part of the treatment that works well for one child may not work as well—or at all—for another. *Inconvenient, but true.* As parents, our job is to find the balance that works for our one-of-a-kind, one-in-a-million kid.

ACTION LIST

When your doctor determines that your child is ready, and if it is something with which you feel comfortable and feel may benefit your child, begin standard chelation therapy using the chelating agent your doctor has recommended.

Monitor closely, with your doctor, the tests of your child's urine and stool samples to determine the effectiveness of this therapy.

Most importantly, continue to keep good records of the improvements you see in your child's behaviors as they are probably the most significant measure of any therapy's effectiveness.

During chelation, you may find that obsessive-compulsive behaviors dwindle and that stimming is nearly gone. You'll also find that your child is taking renewed pleasure in normal play activities, that he's more confident in initiating play with other children, and is making new strides in his attempts—and his abilities—to fit in. You'll likely also find that your child is able to enjoy engaging in quiet activities, such as reading and coloring.

**Monitor closely, with your doctor, the results of other tests
your doctor is running to regularly measure the nutrients your
child's body has available to it.**
Make adjustments in your child's supplement schedule as necessary
to replace any nutrients, especially minerals, that are being lost during the chelation process.

Remove toxins from your home.
Of all of the tasks I've talked about in these action lists at the end of
every chapter, this one will likely be the most daunting. It has to do
with the everyday products and furnishings in our homes that are
toxic to us and our children. Sometimes, it can seem as if there are
so many of them that we can never have home environments that
are truly free from toxins and altogether healthy. We can. But it will
probably take you time to replace all of the unhealthy things you've
been living with, and it will not be inexpensive. So don't try to do it
all at once. Work within the family budget and know that every
small change you make along the way is a much larger improvement
than what it might seem to be out of the context of the complete
wholesome environment you are trying to create. Consider starting
with these suggestions.

- When you bring home your dry cleaning, before you hang it
  in the closet, remove and recycle the plastic hanging bags and
  let it air out, preferably outside if possible, to reduce the level
  of dry-cleaning chemicals you wear directly against your
  skin.
- Have all amalgam (silver-looking, mercury-containing) fillings removed from your family's mouths by a dentist competent in the procedure and replace them with white composite
  material. You'll likely be alarmed, as I was, to see compounds
  that came out of your mouth being moved directly into a bio-
  hazard waste container, but you will likely also be amazed at
  the soaring new levels of focus and concentration you'll be

able to maintain when these amalgams are removed and no longer leaching mercury vapors into your system. If your child has braces, or will be needing braces, seek out an orthodontist who is skilled in working with the new, nonmetallic materials. They are slightly more expensive and sometimes more prone to issues like brackets falling off or breakage, but I think they are worth it.

- As I suggested in Visit #1's Action List, you should, by now, have used up all of your chemical-based cleaning fluids and replaced them with organic or citrus-based solvents. Start to focus on larger items in your home. As your family budget allows, think about replacing carpets with tile or carefully selected green hardwood floors, and upholstered pieces that leach toxins with ones made with a more organic approach. A good, though alarming, website to use to start determining which products and furnishings in your house are toxic is ewg.org. The Environmental Working Group is diligent in documenting the seemingly endless sources of toxicity to which we expose ourselves. It can be overwhelming at first visit, but if you individualize your approach to fit your family's budget and capacity for change, you can make great strides in cleaning up the world in which your family lives.

- If you are vaccinating your children, require that your doctor inject them only with thimerosal-free vaccines. Be aware that "thimerosal free" can be similar to "fat free"—that is, the vaccine may be labeled "thimerosal free" but could still contain traces of mercury in the vaccine. The difference between "thimerosal free" and "fat free" is that traces of fat are unlikely to immediately and significantly impact your body's health. The traces of mercury left in a "thimerosal free" vaccine are sufficient to significantly impair immune function. This is well documented by work published in the medical literature from the University of California–Davis in 2006 and from the University of California–Irvine in 2007. Thimerosal, which is by weight approximately 49 percent mercury, has been used routinely in vaccines as a preservative. In affluent countries, such as the United States and those in the European Union, thimerosal is being phased out, as packaging vaccines in single-dose vials eliminates the need for the preservative. What matters, however, is not your geography or the year in which your child is being vaccinated, but the year the vaccine he was or is being injected with was *manufactured*. Cross-check the vial in your physician's office against the list provided at www.vaccinesafety.edu/thi-table.htm to make sure the vaccine was manufactured after thimerosal phase out began.

If you haven't already done so, join an autism support group.
My local favorite, in my home near Jacksonville, Florida, is www.healautismnow.org. Nationally, there are many, and there is not enough room to list all of the fabulous groups out there, but www.autism.org, www.talkaboutcuringautism.org, www.nationalautism association.org, www.unlockingautism.org, and www.generation rescue.org are just a few that understand and support the biomedical approach and the concept that autism is a treatable disease from which patients can recover. They are not just about raising awareness; they are about finding solutions and ending this epidemic.

Find a group in which you're comfortable. These groups are wonderful places to do more than just get tasty new GFCF recipes—although that is another advantage of joining them. These groups are places to go to for advice and support, or even just to vent to people who know intimately what you are feeling because they are going through it or they have gone through the same processes as you. Become an active part of one of these communities, because they are, above all, places to share and celebrate the achievement of milestones with others who understand exactly the thrill of every new word your child gains, every new day without stimming, every new morning with a good, solid, regular poop. They are good places to turn to in the quest for balance.

HAVE WE DONE ALL THAT WE CAN FOR THIS CHILD?

In the quiet moments when I worry about how sick my children's bodies are, I wonder what their future holds. I have good reason to hope that the little guys who are coming through now will do pretty well over time, with enough support. They are clearly going to have language, and become participating members of society. Many or even most of them should be able to attend college, and hopefully sustain relationships well enough to have a wedding to which they can invite me.

I do worry, though, about the long-term health of these children. I suspect that we will find they are much more ill than any of us ever suspected. There is a family for whom I care across several generations that illustrates this beautifully.

Poppa Pete has a now-teenaged, autistic grandchild in my practice who has, with several long hard years of work, done extremely well. Pete himself was a successful businessman who worked through lunch for years, munching on tuna fish sandwiches, and came to me as a candidate, according to himself and his family, for a starring role in the remake of the movie *Grumpy Old Men*. We did minimal blood work and started an elemental version of what I had done with his grandson. In just a few weeks, his blood pressure, his cholesterol, and his demeanor were remarkably improved. So much so that everyone in his family was stopping me in the office, in the grocery store, at local events, all to tell me that when Poppa's happy, everyone's happy, and they were all happy. It was relatively easy to restore his mood, his behavior, and his health.

For some of the children, even though we manage to normalize so much of their behaviors and their bodies seem so much healthier, it can take years before we can successfully begin to withdraw support. As we continue to research and continue to monitor what my patient's bodies are doing, we are finding an alarming trend to developing autoimmune disease, and our kids are manifesting more than one simultaneously.

The other thing that is certain is that we don't yet know how puberty is going to influence this disease process; early indicators are that it's very difficult and no easier. Nor do we know how the disease is going to influence puberty. Many of our children appear to be starting the process of going through puberty very young.

The thing that lurks in the back of my mind is that when a body is disrupted for a long time, it seems to have an increased propensity to malignancy. This is absolutely an unacceptable possibility to me, and always sends me scurrying back to my books, back to the biochemical pathways looking for answers. Surely if we all work hard enough and fast enough—and by "we" I mean clinicians like myself and autistic kids and their parents, as well as scientists and researchers who are tuned in to biomedical realities—my kids can spend their adulthood managing wellness instead of dealing with sickness. Given the uphill struggle to find acceptance for a biomedical treatment model with proven efficacy, you can see why people in the autism community are sometimes so desperate.

But there are two kinds of people in the world—the kind who see the glass as half full, and the kind who see the glass as half empty, optimist and pessimist. I suspect I have always had a natural abundance of optimism, because I am the half-full kind of person. That is why, when it comes to the ongoing management of autism, I encourage my patients' parents to look down the long road of life and think of the ongoing care their child will likely need not as managing the child's *disease,* but as managing his *health.*

We all need to manage our health, right? Whether that means that an already robustly healthy woman manages to stay that way by eating a lot of fruits and vegetables and doing regular workouts, or your dad manages his high blood pressure with a good diet and a regular prescription drug, or your sister manages her diabetes by eating right and giving herself daily insulin injections, or I manage a bad back with an evening yoga class three or four times a week—we are all engaged in the ongoing process of taking care of ourselves. Managing autism may take a bit more planning, and a bit more perseverance, but in the end, managing the physical illness doesn't have to be, with proper early care, a whole lot different from keeping high blood pressure or a bad back in check.

Managing the health of an autistic child can be easier for some families than for others. Take Aaron, my South African patient. He was diagnosed early, at two years of age, and his parents acted aggressively to get him into biomedical treatment and on the path to recovery. Because of this early and aggressive intervention, Aaron will likely go on to lead a very typical kind of life—he has every chance of graduating from adolescence with no more than his fair share of adolescent bumps, going on to college, establishing a satisfying career, getting married, and having his own family.

That's what I work for, you know—wedding invitations. Biomedical treatment for autism is evolving—we're still in the early stages of learning how to fight this epidemic—but we are on the cutting edge of the cutting edge of an emerging body of science, so I have every reason to hope for those wedding invitations from my former patients to arrive in the mail someday. We have no way of knowing at this point how Aaron will have to manage his health throughout his life. I suspect he may always have to monitor his diet for gluten and casein—the way people who are allergic to peanuts, for instance, or who are lactose intolerant have to manage their diets—and he may always need more than the typical level of support from vitamin and mineral supplements, or even enzymes or probiotics. But rather than ending up in an institution, wearing a helmet so that he won't injure himself, as a mistaken case of psychiatric illness, Aaron is moving into the productive and fulfilling life that was always possible before he got sick. Aaron's progress is thrilling for me, and not least because I am the sort of person who adores going to weddings.

But, as it is with all of my patients, while Aaron is going through his childhood and teenage years, there is always the single question on my mind: Have we done all that we can for this child? It's a question that will be easier to answer for some children than for others, but there are some fiery hoops that can be fairly common along the way, and I want to tell you about some of them.

KYLE

Kyle is a curious, happy seven-year-old with a shock of red hair and abundant freckles. Except for some still-apparent stimming when he gets excited and some lingering problems with concentration in school, he could easily be taken for a typical kid. Interestingly, Kyle's mother, Mo, is a head-turner. She is a well-turned-out business-woman, a high-powered glamour girl who pushes a strand of immaculately coiffed hair back into place with a manicured hand before taking out the exquisite black leather book she uses as Kyle's recovery journal to tell me about his progress. Every once in a while, through the course of our appointment, she glances down at the vibrating Blackberry in her lap to see who's trying to reach her now, mostly ignoring the people who would like to interrupt us, but, infrequently, throwing me a little grimace to let me know this is a call she has to take. At these times I nod at her—"Go ahead"—because I know things about Kyle and Mo that most people would not easily gather just from looking at this striking woman and her curious, happy son: Mo is a struggling single mother trying to do the best she can for her son in the absence of both emotional and financial support from her ex-husband. She is also, like so many in the post-bubble economy, anxious about job security and losing the health benefits that right now come with her job.

Part and parcel of the job of taking medical care of autistic kids is being an advocate for them. Hence my work with the foundation I helped to establish, HEAL!; the travel I do to educate other doctors in biomedical treatment; and the interventions I perform between patients and their insurers.

It's routine for me or my office manager to write letters to or get on the phone with insurance providers to medically validate a patient's claim. As an entity, biomedical intervention, no matter how medically appropriate, is not yet willingly covered by most insurers, but many of the individual *portions* of the treatment are currently sanctioned by the established medical world. I see doing all I can to help my patients' parents be reimbursed for these treatments as part of the work of my office and my office staff. Don't be afraid to ask your doctor to write that letter or make that phone call that will provide your insurer with the additional paperwork it needs to understand that your claim is indeed a covered medical benefit and should be reimbursed.

What is reimbursable will, of course, vary from insurer to insurer, so it isn't practical to go into much detail here about what might be specific to any one policy. You should, however, pursue every opportunity for reimbursement, and your doctor should be a partner to you in this effort. You should, as well, talk to your doctor about programs beyond standard medical insurance that might be available in your state to help you with the financial aspects of treatment—that is, helping to fund the purchase of any special equipment, transportation to and from doctor or therapy appointments, and assistance with child care. Though your physician may not be able to provide direct support in these areas, increasingly they will be able to help point you to individuals and groups who are devoted to getting families started on this path. Once again, I urge you to become involved with an autism support group and to take advantage of all of the resources and wisdom they have to offer.

Mo's healthcare worries often made her life seem tenuous. So there was one piece of information she had to report to me that made us both break out in big, happy smiles: she had just received confirmation that Kyle was eligible for a personal care assistant (PCA) through a state-run program. The PCA would accompany Kyle to school for four hours each day, helping Kyle to stay focused on his classroom lessons and his homework, and would also work with Kyle for eight hours on the weekends.

For some autistic kids, the level of interaction they need to keep them engaged is nearly constant in order for them to get incrementally better. Until now, this constant engagement had been left entirely to Kyle's teacher during school hours and to Mo alone when Kyle was not in school. The PCA was going to make a tremendous difference in both of their lives—the backup of the PCA would allow the teacher to run a more integrated classroom, benefiting not just Kyle but all of her students, and Mo would be able to concentrate with more freedom and less guilt on the job she desperately needed to keep to support herself and Kyle. Mo expressed her relief to me in this way: "It's like we've been handed a get-out-of-jail-free card!"

But Mo's relief didn't end there. "The PCA," she told me, "is a *guy!*" Now, rather than being under the supervision of his mom or his female teacher all day, Kyle was going to get a male role model in his life. "He'll get to do 'guy things'!" Mo told me, so happy for her son she actually laughed.

It wasn't Kyle's dad who would be teaching him about these guy things, as, ideally, it might have been. But by pursuing every avenue that was available to her, Mo found a guy to come into Kyle's life at just the age when he was really starting to need one.

Explore every avenue that's available for you to get help too. Pick your doctor's brain for advice on programs she would recommend. Enlist her as your advocate.

CHARLIE

Charlie is a little guy you might describe as "all boy"—rough and tumble, not immovable as he'd been when I first started to see him and, then, when you did try to move him, inconsolable about it, but still, at four years old, inappropriately physically assertive. He'd started to make some verbal progress, but it was still only his parents and I who, for the most part, had the patience to get hold of him, slow him down, and ask him to repeat himself so that we could understand what it was he wanted to say. His poops still had a gray tint to them, and there was huge volume whenever he had a bowel movement. Now he was in my office because he had another ear infection. I closed my eyes for a moment, knowing what I had to do: write him a prescription for antibiotics and tell his earnest parents to brace themselves for another possible regression.

Biomedical intervention, as I've tried to make very clear in these pages, does not provide instantaneous answers. Our children don't magically recover from their allergies, their bowel problems, or their reflux disease after the first month or so of treatment. The inflammation they suffer may require a more aggressive approach than usual. Their yeast problem may prove to be very stubborn. The experience of chronic infections doesn't just stop, but, like Charlie's, may demand that we once again experiment with changing the child's diet, changing his probiotics, slowing down the dosage of a chelating agent, or speeding up hyperbaric treatments. Each individual child will usually have at least one very individual biochemical issue we will have to overcome with modified doses of either vitamin C, iodine, lysine, GABA, antihistamines, antifungals, antiparasitics, or anti-inflammatories. In Charlie's case, it was antibiotics to address his chronic earaches and infections.

Charlie's parents—his dad, an imposing Latino patriarch who adored his family, and his mother, who often let her husband speak for her but only because she was still learning to speak English— and I looked at each other warily. Charlie's progress, to date, had been uneven. His small body had been badly compromised, and his response to treatment was, accordingly, slow and erratic. He still had to be keenly supervised whenever he left the house or he might "escape"—take off at a gallop down a strange street or through a shopping mall, causing his mom to panic and sometimes enlist store security, or even the police, to help her pursue him. His dad had yet to fix the hole in the dining room wall where Charlie had kicked it after his *last* bout with antibiotics had gone badly. We were all aware that giving him antibiotics again could be a bad tipping point.

But we had no choice.

I wrote the prescription, and we hugged each other, and I asked Charlie's mom to call me the next day and let me know how he was doing.

Your child may respond to treatment beautifully at first, and he may—like Aaron—be one of those kids who very rarely have any sort of a setback and simply sail through recovery. But, realistically, you have to prepare yourself for setbacks of the sort Charlie and his parents faced. A big part of getting through the almost inevitable impediments is the relationship you establish with your doctor. You want to find a doctor who you are going to feel comfortable calling the next day—and the day after that and, if need be, the day after that—to respond with changes in a prescription and advice about tweaking dosages until you have been able to bring your child back from her setback and are, once again, ready to move forward in recovery.

In the meantime, I gave Charlie's dad the web address of a company, one of many I'm sure, that makes gluten-, casein-, and soy-free, but not organic (we can't have it all) temporary tattoos (www.wwwtemporarytattoos.com) and told them to order in a supply with Charlie's name, his illness, and their cell phone numbers on it. They could put a fresh one on him every day after his morning bath, so in case he decided to escape again during this course of antibiotics, they could rest a little easier while mall security helped them search for him under the clothing racks where he liked to hide.

Charlie's parents did, indeed, get the tattoos. These temporary tattoos are one of the tricks I recommend all my parents keep up their sleeves, especially when the family is going on vacation, away from the child's familiar territory. And Charlie's mom did call me every day to report on how Charlie was doing on his antibiotics—which was consistently *great*. As it turned out, the antibiotics *were* a tipping point for Charlie, but of the good kind. For the first time, Charlie made it through a course of antibiotics without regressing. We had hit a new plateau in his healing process. For the first time we could move onward—upward—without having to take a step or two backward first.

CHRISTOPHER

DANI: Hey, Mom what do you call it when you attack someone who insults you?

JULIE: I don't know. What do you call that, Dani?

DANI: An offensive tackle.

In our football-loving household, I suppose that if my daughter was going to start making up jokes, I shouldn't have been surprised that they would revolve around our favorite game. What was remarkable was that Dani's sense of humor was awakening, emerging from the fog of autism.

"Let me tell you about the cute things he's starting to do," one of my parents told me during an appointment. "He's getting up on the bed and jumping on it while I'm trying to make it. At first I was annoyed with him, and then I saw this sly little grin on his face. It was a joke! He was trying to be funny! I laughed so hard, it was so funny, it was so beautiful, seeing him make a joke again!"

"You gotta hear this," another parent insists. "The other night my husband was reading the newspaper, and all of a sudden, Erik walks over and turns the lamp off. My husband looks up, like, Who did that? And Erik's standing there, giggling like a little devil."

These stories make me laugh right along with the parents—it absolutely feels like one of the most joyous events in life when our kids, formerly so blank, their expressions so flat, start wisecracking again. When they start to awaken.

"He sat right down and did his math worksheets when he got home from school *all by himself.* He figured it out—school, then homework, then playtime. He's starting to get the structure, you know, of how life's supposed to work. He's learning to be an honest-to-God student."

"She asked if she could go out for basketball. A *team* sport. I was like, Yes, yes, yes!"

"If I won't let him change the radio station in the car he just shrugs at me and turns to his dad and asks again. He's learning to divide and conquer." Even the lessons we ordinarily wouldn't want our kids to learn can feel like progress, because these lessons are signs that they are becoming typical kids. These kids, who might have been, even just a few years ago, consigned to a lifetime in an institution, are starting to take part in life again.

One of the tools I recommend to parents to help nurture this growth of interest is one of the listening programs.

One such program was developed by Dr. Alfred Tomatis to help students who were struggling academically, had difficulties with language, or who had problems remembering what they had heard. In the years since the therapy was developed, listening programs have also proven to be effective for children with articulation problems, sound sensitivity, attention deficits, poor physical coordination, low social skills, low energy or low confidence levels, and sleep problems—all issues that can be a part of autism.

The program works by literally exercising the tiny muscles in the ear, which helps to establish stronger multisensory pathways in the brain. Through the use of classical music played and recorded in unique ways, so that each instrument is a discrete yet distinct sound, both hemispheres of the brain synchronize and begin to work together. The music is highly organized, in patterns that resonate in the brain, to effect what scientists call the *plasticity factor*, the brain's natural capacity to change its structure in response to experience and stimulation coming to it from the outside.

Each of the listening programs has its merits. One of my favorites because of its combined quality and affordability is The Listening Program. The program consists of a series of CDs that are to be played through headphones—either one of a number of recommended high-quality brands, or through a special "bone conduction" set that allows the sounds on the CDs to actually penetrate through bone resonance for a different sort of processing by the brain.

One of the first people to whom I recommended The Listening Program was Christopher's mother. Christopher was a perfectly charming-looking six-year-old who was progressing well physically, but only plodding obediently through school and family life. He seemed to have no spark. Nothing interested him. Nothing turned him on and made him light up.

His mother called the day after Christopher used The Listening Program for the first time. "When the session was over, he immediately got up and went to his room and started to strum his guitar." Christopher's parents had bought the guitar because music was the one thing that had seemed to make him turn his head and pay attention, and they would have tried anything to see again childhood's look of wonder and discovery on Christopher's face. Now, after just one session with The Listening Program, for the first time ever, he'd actually picked up the guitar. "Something," his mother told me, in awe, "is awakening."

JACK AND DARIUS

Jack and Darius have both been my patients for about four years; they both came early to my specialized practice.

Jack is twenty years old, with deep brown eyes, and when you look into them you can see the kid who's supposed to be walking across campus, one arm slung around his girlfriend's shoulder, a basketball tucked under the other, laughing, learning, making his life's plans.

But that scene may never happen in Jack's life. He was 16 before we began biomedical intervention; his body is very profoundly damaged. He stims almost constantly, stiffening himself and holding his breath, and he asks repeatedly for his mother to clean his eyeglasses or give him a squeeze. He talks easily, but he's really only completely articulate when he's outraged, which he often is. His little brother has recently gone off to college, and Jack acknowledges this departure with the refrain, "I'm a dummie." The frustration in his words is palpable.

Darius, on the other hand, is eight years old, an early catch, a little boy who began biomedical intervention at the age of four and had made enough progress to be doing passably well in a regular classroom. As it turned out, however, Darius is a bit of a genius. His mother caught him up past his bedtime, in his room, working algebra problems for fun.

"Where did you learn to do that?" she asked him, more amazed at the algebra solutions sitting in front of him than angry he was up so late.

Darius had been walking by his older sister while she sat at the dining room table every evening doing her algebra homework and thought the problems looked like fun.

"My God," his mother sighed to me, "here we were, trying to teach him to *count* and he can do *algebra!* How was I supposed to know that?"

I can't answer Darius's mother's larger question—How was she supposed to know?—except to say that as our children progress through the treatment process and grow older, we need to be aware that often autistic kids possess "pockets" of knowledge we can't suspect but should be on the lookout for anyway. As the lack of sight will often force the other senses of a blind person to become more acute, so it seems that when one part of the brain doesn't work well, another part will compensate by working in an exceptional way. It seems that our kids often demonstrate—if we know enough to let them do it—truly exceptional skill in fields such as math, science, and engineering.

These amazing pockets can be found even in kids who have been suffering as long term and profoundly as Jack.

"You're stimming," Jack's mother tells him.

"Yes," Jack agrees and obediently stops, and his mother and I continue our discussion until Jack interrupts again. "Clean," he demands, taking off his eyeglasses and holding them out toward his mother.

"I just did that, Jack. If you want your glasses to be clean, you'll have to do it yourself."

"Yes," Jack tells her, disappointed, but he dutifully polishes the lenses himself, using the bottom hem of his T-shirt. "Squeeze," he orders, and his mother rises to give him one. He's obviously agitated about something.

"Words," Jack had insisted earlier during this appointment until we understood that he was approving the discussion his mother and I were having about restarting his methyl-B_{12} shots and the positive effect that might have on his ability to use language. His parents had given him the shots until about a year earlier, but the small amount of improvement he'd made while on them hadn't impressed his father, and they'd stopped.

So I'd asked him, "Do you want your words back?"

"Yes!" he'd cheered, and relaxed back in his chair, at ease for the moment. Understood.

Now Jack's mother and I were talking about how much Jack liked it when she read to him. But something about the discussion was bothering him.

"Do you like it when your mom reads to you?" I asked him.

"Yes!"

"But you're upset about something?"

"Yes!"

But what?

"What kinds of books do you two read together?" I asked his mother.

"Well"—she shrugged—"you know, readers. Primers. Things Jack can understand, and maybe if I can point the words out to him as I'm saying them, and repeat them often enough, he'll learn to read a few of them..."

Aha. I had a hunch.

"Jack?"

"Yes?"

"What kinds of books do you want your mom to read to you?"

Jack's reply was extraordinary, and articulated as was no other word he'd spoken to us that day, slowly and carefully. "Architecture."

"Architecture!" His mother was stunned.

As stunned as I suppose I might have been if I didn't work with autistic kids every day. If I didn't regularly see the evidence that a highly developed math and engineering skill set was linked somehow to this syndrome.

"You want your mother to read you books about architecture, Jack?" I asked to clarify.

"Yes!" His relief was enormous as he once again sank back in his chair, understood.

As your child progresses through his treatment plan, make sure not to underestimate the skills she may well be acquiring and becoming able to use. Even if he is not yet reading himself, try to read to him at least at the grade level he would be at if he were developing typically. And always—always—keep an eye out for signs that he's got a pocket of knowledge he's aching to share with you and develop, but might not be able just yet to tell you about.

THE LONGEST MARATHON

DANI II

This is the hardest part of the book to write. That's because what I have to say is so very personal. As I was confidently dotting all the i's in the final drafts of my chapters, something happened that threw my world into chaos: my beautiful, now ten-year-old autistic daughter, Dani, began having seizures.

Those of us who live and work with autistic children are altogether too well acquainted with our worlds being thrown into chaos, but Dani had never had a seizure before. I had cared for many a seizing child during my training, but never had I personally experienced the utter terror that overtakes a parent when her child seizes. "I'm here with you," I whispered urgently to her. "Hold on," I commanded. "Breathe," I prayed, though like all parents before me who have witnessed their child seizing, I was not breathing myself. But I had learned the language of this new crisis.

I have likened raising an autistic child to running a marathon, but what we parents know is that sometimes, every few miles, we run into a roadblock, a hurdle to clear, a fiery hoop we have to jump through. First, we start to get our child's fragile GI tract and immune system normalized by getting the child—and often our whole family—accustomed to a whole new way of eating and cooking. We keep meticulous records in order to find the exact balance of nutritional supplements, probiotics, and enzymes that will further strengthen our child. We kill yeast. We infuse our child with glutathione. We sleep with them cuddled next to us in hyperbaric chambers. We chelate. Like Dani, the child gets better, regresses, then gets better again, ultimately improving in some ways small or large at every step. Perhaps, as in my family, we are fortunate and the child regains lost IQ points, succeeds at school, and tentatively but truly steps into the life of a typical child.

In her preteen years, as Dani grew again into the bright, gifted little girl she'd been before her regression, I had good medical reason to hope she might be spared some of the fiery hoops I knew could very well be looming around the next bend of our long race. Having a child who is on the older side of the epidemic wave of autism, I am required to try to stay one step ahead of emerging research, so I knew what might be coming our way. I held my breath, not daring to hope even as the days sped by so uneventfully. I knew that it was not uncommon for autistic children to experience precocious puberty—and I knew it was also not uncommon that as these children reach their preteen years and their hormones begin to assert themselves, their biochemistry will once again be thrown out of whack by raging adolescence. This is, at least in part, probably what happened to Dani in February 2009.

Watching my daughter, holding her, and praying for her while she seized brought every bit of my anger back to the surface. I raged at the forces that had aligned to make my daughter ill. It was powerless rage, and during that first seizure, it spewed from me like so much vomit, alternating in breaths with the prayer for this nightmare to stop, for time to go back and erase this new chapter from Dani's life. In the days that followed, my grief was palpable. My head knew that the practical, productive thing to do was to keep focused on recovery—but my heart knew that the rage was cleansing, an integral part of my own healing. Later, at the moment I allowed my rage to surface again, Dani was home and safe again, and I was out of town. I was with one of my football players, trying to have a bite to eat while we were both on the road in the same city—he to do some off-season training, and me to give a lecture about biomedical intervention.

My football player raged with me—or, I might describe what happened more accurately by saying that he raged *for* me. You see, as sometimes will happen with patients, the football player and his family had become good friends with me and my family—and Dani had become a stand-out favorite of his.

I won't dispute that part of the reason for Dani's charmingly evident crush on the guy is just that he is a huge human being; Dani, I believe, feels particularly safe walking alongside this giant, holding on to his hand, knowing he would keep her safe from anything in this world. It's odd that they should actually be able to do that, hold hands—Dani is so much smaller than he is. I'm sometimes amazed that their hands can reach each other's, but they do. Whenever he and his fiancé come to the house for dinner, there is always time for him to curl up with Dani on the sofa in our family room. He looks over the schoolwork she shows off to him, or he reads with her while the rest of us finish preparing dinner, Dani cuddled up beside him, an arm draped over his shoulder and her fingers rubbing against the grain of the rough five o'clock shadow on his shaved head.

Now, just the two of us over dinner, this extraordinary young man was giving me an incredible gift: he was taking on some of my anger for me. He, too, was insulted and outraged on Dani's behalf. When someone takes on your anger, an amazing thing happens—you are left with little choice but to let it go. When the load you are carrying feels like a ton of bricks in a handcart you're trying to pull up a steep hill all by yourself, and someone comes along and offers to lighten it, you're relieved, grateful. You can go back to hauling what's left to you with a little more energy, a little more sanity, a little less pain.

And here is where I find God is in all of this, inevitably waiting to soothe me through my trouble.

I know that there are people who have a hard time reconciling how a person of science can also be a person of faith. They think that scientific reason in some way minimizes, or even negates, the yearning for the spiritual. Perhaps even more to the point, some people may wonder how a family running that marathon with autism may not rail against or abandon a Creator who could deal their child such an unfair blow.

This is a question many siblings of children with autism have asked, sometimes silently communicated in their resentment, and sometimes so obviously answered in their endless patience as they teach and model for their siblings. We, as parents, have no idea, I suspect, how hard their row is to hoe sometimes, for they are left to answer the unkindnesses dished out by their peers when our adult ears are not present to hear. I try to address this by teaching them what I taught my fabulous older son, Matthew, so many years ago. "When someone makes fun of, or is unkind to, your sister or to you because of this thing called autism, you try to teach them a little about autism. If that doesn't work, then you tell them this: 'God must have thought an awful lot more of me than He did of you, because He trusted me, not you, with one of His very special children.' There's just no way for anyone to answer that, son. Then walk away and let them think a bit." I find it helps siblings to feel and know how very special they are, and including them in the recovery helps them to know they are not alone, that they are part of the team.

So I know that God is very much a part of the team as well. And in the very miracle of biochemistry itself, and in the human capacity to learn about it and find within it ways to help and to heal, I, as a scientist, find a perfect basis for faith. This faith includes the unassailable understanding that God gives me only what I can handle; and the more He gives me, the more He trusts me. Sometimes—to, however presumptuously, paraphrase Mother Teresa—I wish He didn't trust me so much. But I surely know that He trusts autistic kids like Dani even more, and I can often take my lessons directly from them. "I'm here Mommy, it's okay," Dani tells me now after a seizure, when she hears the question in my voice and feels the questioning in my face and my spirit. If she is so okay, how can I not be too? How can I stay inside my sorrow or my anger and not try to find that thing God has entrusted me with this time?

My son and husband were with Dani and me at the local emergency room following her first seizure. After a seizure, a series of neurological tests have to be performed to eliminate new concerns and to help guide future treatment. The problem with having to go to the hospital is that I have made quite a name for myself. Years ago, when I started down this path, I was regarded by the medical establishment as one of those doctors who engages in the "pseudoscience" of biochemical intervention. Over the years, though, many of my peers have seen the undeniable results in some of their patients and have come to see the validity of this approach to autism. My grief as a mother in the emergency room would be compounded by the frustration of encountering, in all likelihood, a whole host of medical professionals who would not merely reject the efficacy of Dani's treatment out of hand, but who would also—even though they had no clue what they were talking about—be patronizing about it.

At the hospital, we were seen by one of the new residents. The resident might have introduced himself, but I don't remember his name, only that he was young and that, as he examined Dani, he did not speak to her. He listened only perfunctorily when she tried to talk to him and gave a cursory listen to her heart as he asked me about her medical history.

At this point in time, Dani's medical history is a dissertation, of course, and as I talked about her autism and the treatment for it, and as Dani added her own details about her diet and supplement program, I could see the look on the resident's face begin to change. I knew that look; I had seen it so many times: this mother is one of those crazies who think that autism is a toxicity problem.

The funny thing was, even as I kept on talking in what was clearly rational, medical language, the resident kept that "she's a nut" distance on his face—he had stopped paying attention. Since he didn't take a social history, he didn't ask what I did for a living, and I was just perverse enough not to clue him in. When he'd finished what he thought was a sufficient history and physical, he simply got up to leave the room. I took my rising fury at what I knew he was thinking and tried to salvage some thread of communication between us. I turned calmly to Dani.

"You know what, Dani?" I asked her as he walked toward the door.

"What, Mommy?"

"That doctor thinks Mommy's a whacko."

The resident turned around then. He said, "Pretty much," and when he left the room, he closed the door behind him.

It took me about 20 seconds to decide to use the endless waiting time for something positive. I pulled out my cell phone and called BJ up at Project Chance. BJ is an animal trainer who works with lots of differently abled people to match them with service dogs. It was time to get serious about an autism service dog for Dani. We had been talking about it at home and knew that the tremendous relationships our children were forging with their dogs were often life changing. The good news, on that awful night in the emergency room, was that there were some three-week-old puppies, and BJ would reserve one for Dani, pending the interview and evaluation of our family as a good candidate for success. BJ promised me that our puppy would be wonderful for all of us. "Especially for the moms, Julie. The dogs are a mother's helper in so many ways." As she spoke, it became just a little bit easier to imagine Dani sleeping in her own room at night—as long as there was a dog, a guardian angel, to call me if Dani needed me.

About 45 minutes later, one of the old-time ER doctors, Mike, walked into the room. Mike had taken care of Dani on a couple of the occasions on which we had visited the hospital when she was much younger and had had asthma problems, but that had been so many years ago I was sure he didn't remember us. What he did remember was that I am a doctor too, and a pediatrician at that. He listened respectfully as I again laid out Dani's medical history before him—the fact that she was fine, and then suddenly she was not fine, losing her language, all of her accelerated reading skills, and her social graces at age four, and that then, through biomedical intervention, she'd relearned everything, been labeled as gifted, and mainstreamed, and that now she was a growing preteen and her biochemistry must be in an uproar again, triggering this seizure . . .

Mike listened and—here's the fun part—*so did the resident.* Chastened, I suspect, by the paperwork identifying me as a physician that he'd looked at *after* he'd left the room, the resident had, quietly, returned to our examining room and stood listening to the discussion Mike and I were having about Dani's illness. The look on his face was a little different on this, his second go around in our room.

Throughout the talk that Mike and I were having, the resident didn't say a word. After Mike had ordered the neurological tests we'd come for—the CT scan we were going to have done that night and the EEG we were scheduling for a few days later (because in order for an EEG to be accurate you have to wait for several days after a seizure to do it)—and the resident had really heard all we had to say, he simply got up and left again.

I suspect that it was really hard for that resident to come back into the room—it probably felt like he was eating humble pie. But something had moved him to come back to the room and hear the parts of Dani's story he'd missed because he'd so immediately made up his mind about us and our course of treatment. I'll always hope that he came back not because he had to, but because something had made him question the rhetoric he'd been taught in medical school that told him I was wrong about the biomedical model. Perhaps something had opened his mind, and maybe his heart, enough for him to stop clinging for a moment to what he thought he knew and admit new ideas and fresh evidence. Being a young resident, maybe only novelty had compelled him to come back and listen. So many of the older doctors go home wondering, after the fact, about something I said or something they saw, and they never call, no matter how many times I invite them to do just exactly that. It was the "old dog/new trick" problem. "Young man," I prayed silently as Dani and I waited for her test results, "I don't know your name, but I pray for you, that your mind and your heart will continue to open. That maybe you will have been touched just enough by Dani's story to continue to wonder about all the things you do not know, and you will go on to find not just the easy answers, but the correct answers and, in doing so, you will become the very best doctor you can be. This is what I pray for you."

A few days later, Dani and I were back at the hospital clinic for the rest of her neurological tests. Despite all my efforts to reach out to the doctors in the neurology department over the years, my methods usually have been met with, at the least, polite resistance, and at the worst, outright hostility directed toward my patients seeking help with the management of seizures. The feedback these doctors have given to our mutual patients usually contradicts many of my own recommendations. These doctors and I work together under a sort of uneven détente, so for me, the hospital clinic is a place where subtle tension always lurks just beneath the surface. The doctors know that I am always on the edge on their turf, waiting to call out any one of them who insists that autism is a psychiatric disorder rather than a physical illness. We tread lightly around one another.

But this time, I had to be there. I had no choice. Dani had had two more seizures during her EEG, so there was no choice about her needing a neurological evaluation, and unfortunately for them, she needed it today. Luckily, Arthur, an old friend of mine who happens also to be a neurologist, was willing to step up to the plate that day. His wife and I had once been in practice together and had been good friends—a friendship that had waned over the years, not because we did not care to nurture it but because we were both mothers of young children who required our nurturing. Also, we'd both left our old practice, so between the demands of motherhood and the simple fact that we no longer saw each other at work everyday, we'd fallen out of touch. Still, Arthur and I had known each other for a long time. He knew Dani's history. He didn't even have to look at the paperwork to ask me the crucial question: "So what do you want to do, Julie?"

In addition to being in a place that always made me feel uncomfortably defensive, you see, I also carried the tension of knowing what was coming next. The seizures Dani had had were of two different types—the first was a complex partial seizure and the ones during her EEG were absence seizures, also known as *petit mal*. I knew that without question the indication was to start her on some sort of antiseizure medication—and Arthur knew it too.

Near tears, I said, "I have to, don't I?" still hoping he'd say it wasn't necessary to start her on meds today.

"You really do, she's having unprovoked seizures, Julie." So I breathed, every last vestige of denial yanked out from underneath me; we really were on this road now, and I waited. "Which one?" he asked, meaning, which antiseizure medication was I going to choose?

Antiseizure medications are terrible things. Our kids have historically done very poorly on them because the medications invariably contain an ingredient, or sometimes more than one ingredient, in their formulas that impact negatively on some other aspect—cycle—of our kids' fragile systems.

"I'm not going to give up cognitive function," I replied, because some antiseizure medications can absolutely wipe out cognitive function. "Dani's worked too hard to get that back and I'm not giving it up."

Arthur had nodded. "Then let's rule a few out, and we'll choose based on these two very different types of seizures she's shown us," he told me. "Lamictal," he decided, and he left to go get me some samples of it he had on hand.

What happened in the 15 minutes that followed is a blur. Arthur was in and out of the room, going out to get the Lamictal and bringing it back, coming and going several more times to retrieve his stethoscope, paperwork, and God knows what else, while I fumbled to find the package insert in the Lamictal to read about its ingredients. During one of these trips in and out, one of Arthur's partners entered the room with him. Arthur introduced us. When the partner heard my name, he said, "I believe we have some patients in common, Dr. Buckley"—and he stood looking down at me as I racked my brain trying to remember which patients and what exactly he had said to them about me. It was probably a good thing I couldn't remember at that particular moment.

I was trying to give him the benefit of the doubt, but I was pretty sure I had never experienced such outright condescension from someone I had never met before. Arthur tried to defuse the tension. "Julie and my wife were partners, years ago."

The partner didn't seem to hear him. Instead he mumbled something at me that sounded like, "I'm sure you're just trying to help parents who are absolutely desperate . . ." I knew what he meant—that I was a quack offering hope where there was none—but in another way he was right and had no idea why: my patients' parents were, just like I was, desperate for the medical community to acknowledge and then *act on* what we knew to be true about the treatment and recovery of autistic kids.

But I didn't have the energy to argue with him that evening; my thoughts were totally occupied with the necessity of starting Dani on a frightening new class of drugs and what those drugs might mean to her overall health. I just nodded at him dumbly and went back to looking for the information I was seeking in the fine print of the Lamictal package insert.

Arthur attempted again to keep the meeting cordial, introducing his partner to Dani and telling him why she and I were there.

"Ah," the partner said knowingly, without knowing the first thing about who Dani was and what sort of massive medical history her short life had already generated, "so, we have new onset juvenile epilepsy . . ."

We all sort of continued to nod our heads politely through the awkward conversation. But then I felt my nodding head jerk of its own accord, seize in the middle of the up-and-down motion of a "yes" and start itself going side-to-side, shaking "no." What form of mental block did these guys have? What *was* it that prevented them from sensibly looking at the science that was showing such positive results for our autistic kids?

"No," I said, thinking, even as I spoke, Julie, do *not* unleash your fury on this man who probably intends you no harm, "*No*. It is *not* idiopathic. She was fine, and then she was not fine. This is not idiopathic, it's toxic . . ."

I know I said more, kept talking, but the guy was out of the room in a heartbeat.

Arthur came over and sat down next to me.

I was so angry I was shaking. Tears of anger, tears of frustration, tears of grief threatened to spill over my exhausted eyelids. Still, I held back from taking it out on my old friend Arthur. "I make all of you so uncomfortable," I said.

Arthur looked away and took a deep breath as he found his words. "Julie, I've known you for years. It's okay. I'm good with it."

I let that sink in for a second, then quietly replied, "Well, all right then." And I turned my attention back to hunting for the list of ingredients on the damned package insert. Reading the ingredients on that package insert was the most important task I had to perform anyway. Did it matter, right at that moment, who I made uncomfortable? What was I about to start giving my kid, and how was it going to impact her health? Those were the questions, and they were such scary ones that my hands were still shaking, wrestling with the drug's packaging.

But I couldn't find the list of ingredients. I still don't know whether that was because I was so clumsy in the moment or whether, more likely, it was one of those God moments, but I ended up just squinting at the drug label to see if it contained any important information. And the first thing I saw there was mighty important indeed: Lamictal depresses folate metabolism.

"Arthur, I can't give this to Dani."

Let me say here that Arthur, as a professional courtesy, had fit Dani and me into his schedule on an emergency basis. It was late on a Friday afternoon, and he had stayed at his office only to be able to see Dani. For all of his kindness, he was tired.

"What?" He only just escaped sounding incredulous.

"I mean, Arthur, I'm going to give it to her, I know I have to, but Lamictal depresses folate metabolism—and I'm going to tell you a way around it."

Arthur's look was just plain blank, and I could see him suppressing a sigh, not making the connection.

"Folate metabolism is something our kids have problems with anyway. If they take this drug, it'll make it worse."

Arthur looked even more tired, but he couldn't keep himself from looking interested too, since I had promised a way around the problem.

"This is the exact spot where methyl-B_{12} metabolism breaks down. If their systems can't make methyl-B_{12} then they can't make glutathione, and if they can't make glutathione they can't manage their oxidative stress. Given what Dani's brain has just been through, I can't imagine the amount of glutathione her neurons must need right now."

Arthur was right with me. "So, what do you do about that, considering her body needs the antiseizure med too?"

"Start her on this stuff called CerefolinNAC at the same time as we start the Lamictal." I'd just heard about Cerefolin myself, at a think tank the week before. It was a new prescription-requiring supplement that supports folate metabolism, ironically pioneered by a physician from the hospital next door. Nobody could have blamed Arthur for not knowing about Cerefolin yet, but I couldn't resist the opportunity to give back a little of what I'd been getting at the hospital: "The good news, Arthur, is that it's a prescription drug. That ought to give you some comfort."

Arthur had the grace to laugh. Then, saying, "I wonder if it's on formulary here?" he pulled up the electronic drug list, and there it was. Suddenly, it was real to him. He looked at me and offered quietly, "Well, Julie, you just taught me something."

And as I felt a little bridge beginning to build, I felt the long-shut door maybe—just maybe—begin to open a tad; a little of the anger was replaced with a hint of peace.

It truly is the little children who lead us. In the week since Dani's first seizure, she and I had built two little bridges to the medical establishment. There was a good chance we'd piqued the curiosity of at least one resident and that, if our prayers were answered, he was going to be a better, more compassionate doctor because of it. And hopefully, Arthur was never again going to prescribe a seizure medicine to an autistic kid without at least wondering, if not fully understanding, how the drug might impact the overall health of that child. If we were lucky, he would look, from today forward, at the treatment of autism a little more broadly and take steps—like prescribing Cerefolin along with Lamictal—to mitigate any negative effects.

It was a weird few weeks, that period when Dani started having her seizures. These weren't the only two bridges built. Jerry Kartzinel and I were giving a HEAL!-sponsored talk about biomedical intervention in autism for our local community. We invited folks in the medical establishment we knew were at least intrigued, listening to what we'd had to say through our patients—about 30 all told. It was a talk geared for medical people, heavy on the science, technical slides, reference materials, and statistics from research studies.

Twelve people showed up.

The audience was small, but Jerry and I went ahead with the presentation as if we were talking to the whole world—because we know it is the whole world we will have to enlighten, and neither one of us is afraid of having to repeat ourselves. We'll talk to one person at a time if that's what it takes.

Still, you never really know how your material has been received until a presentation is over and the lights come back up and your audience starts to react. That night, 1 person in our small audience of 12, a psychiatrist, asked, with tears in her eyes, the $64,000 question: *They told us there was no science in this. Why have I never seen this science before?* But it wasn't really a question, it was a howl of enormous dissatisfaction, and the answer didn't matter anyway because she got it. She got that there was some important information about autism she'd been missing in all her years in practice. She understood what the parents of autistic kids and practitioners like myself have been trying to get the established medical community to hear for years.

It had been such a hard, weird few weeks, I could have rushed into the audience and kissed her, but the rest of the audience started to shift in their seats. The rumble of Q-and-A began, and I knew we had at least 1 and maybe 12 new people who would be willing to learn with and from our patients and us—new members of our team.

Angie II

Later during this same time period, late on another Friday afternoon, my last patient of the week came charging into my office and threw her arms around me for the greeting that had become customary between us over the years—a wild big bear hug.

"How is Angie?" I asked her, not realizing exactly how much this now 14-year-old young woman had to report to me.

The bloated, blank-faced little girl who, just four years earlier, had banged her head against any hard surface she could find to try to displace some of the unbearable pain of the physical illness of autism, is now a beautiful teenager with one of the widest, most disarming smiles I've ever seen on anybody, and laughing eyes that just kill me. Sometimes I go back through her files, through all my patients' files, and see the early photographs of them that are stored there, just to realize anew how far these kids have come. Angie still has a few lingering signs that might tip you off that, at one time, she was physically very sick. Her verbal skills aren't perfect; when she speaks, all the sounds are not quite perfectly articulated, and she sounds very much, in fact, as if she has had a hearing impairment and is bravely speaking words she has never actually heard pronounced. And her pinky fingers are very short. Her stalwart mother has just agreed that Angie can be one of the subjects of a new study that will seek to determine the cause of such physical deformities. My bet? Ain't no gene that did that to her fingers. It's the toxins.

But other than these slight lingering problems? The ten-year-old girl who was once headed for a lifetime in an institution for the permanently brain damaged is a lively young teenager chattering to me about the 100 percent she got that afternoon on her science test in the school where she is mainstreamed. Her mother is adding that her project at the science fair won second prize. She is smiling, and shrugging ever so slightly to let me know that, had Angie worked just a little harder, maybe it could have been first place. Angie is playfully ignoring her mother, changing the subject, now telling me about the dance she attended the weekend before—her first school dance!

"Did you go with a boy?" I teased her.

"No," Angie told me quickly, but she drew the word out to let me know that going with a boy to the next dance wasn't totally out of the question.

"Any *certain* boy?" I asked, but her mother was groaning.

"No boys," she insisted. Like any typical mother of any typical young teenager, she was not overly anxious for the dating phase of her daughter's life to begin.

"Well, *maybe* . . . ," Angie demurred. This was clearly a subject that was going to be taken up again at home, Angie asserting her preferences and claiming her own ground.

The whole scene that was taking place in my office would be unbelievable to any doctor still resistant to the biomedical treatment of autism. "Not possible," those sorts of doctors would bluster, meaning that they believe recovery from autism is not possible, and that Angie had not really been autistic at the outset of her treatment, and I'd get my back up—"What, are you blind? Take a look at this child right in front of you and then tell me what didn't work!" I know all this, but right now my heart is too full to admit even one molecule of anger. My heart is dancing, as a matter of fact, and I haven't even heard the real news yet. Angie's mother looked at me slyly. "Go on, Angie, tell Dr. Julie what you told me yesterday."

"What?" Angie answered, thoroughly confused. I imagined this chatterbox had told her mother a great many things between yesterday and this afternoon.

"What you told me about what you want to do when you grow up."

This stops me in my tracks. You see, of all the lingering signs of autism, one of the most distressing to me is that autistic kids have a hard time conceiving of the future. Asking them to make plans, or even what they imagine their plans could be, can be a heartrending experience. Angie had decided what she wanted to be when she grew up?

"Well . . . ," Angie began, as shy as any teenager revealing a secret. "First I'm going to go to Gainesville . . ."

"Going to Gainesville," to high school students in the part of Florida where Angie and I live, means becoming a student at the University of Florida.

College? Angie was planning on college!

"Tell her why you want to go to Gainesville," Angie's mother prodded, in case the answer wasn't self evident.

"To be a Gator," Angie said, and you could just about hear the *Duh* in her answer.

I was still back on Angie planning on college for herself. I sometimes have to remember that I am a doctor and, at least in my own office, I have to maintain a little dignity, because what I wanted to do was to start jumping up and down. What I did though, as calmly as possible, was to ask, "And what are you going to study in college, Angie?"

Here Angie grew silent, though her smile grew even wider.

"Go on, you can tell Dr. Julie," her mother said.

What, indeed, was Angie hoping to be when she grew up?

"A nurse," was what she told me. "And I'm going to come to work for you in your office," she added quickly, with utter confidence.

Angie's mother and I exchanged looks. I'm sure she could see the calculations going on in my mind: Angie was 14 years old, well past her preteen years. There was every possibility that Angie had completely escaped the fiery hoop of raging hormones and seizures. There was every possibility that the future Angie was starting to plan for herself could really happen.

The most sorrowful thing any parent ever has to do is to cross something off his child's list of possibilities.

Typical kids start out with endless options. Now, because of Dani's seizures, there are things that once again have to be crossed off her list—at least temporarily. For now, she can't walk the half block from home to her grandmother's house without supervision. Not until we get her seizures under control. For now, she can't look forward to getting her driver's license. Not until we get this new problem solved. For now, she can't . . . Oh, I don't know—she can't go skydiving!

Not that Dani would go skydiving on a bet, but if she wanted to, right now she couldn't dream of it. That option is closed to her. The sky is no longer the limit. The sky won't be the limit again until her body is fixed. Until I, and all of us who are working to defeat autism, learn to fix and polish and ungum these children's systems—and then teach others how to do it too, convince them that it can be done, that *we are doing it.*

It was truly a long, weird few weeks since Dani had gotten sick again. But she was now safe at home, and she hadn't had another seizure in nearly three days. One young resident was likely to no longer passively accept the party line about autism. One doctor had learned how to prescribe medicine so that in the process of helping our kids, it wasn't also hurting them. One attendee at the lecture Jerry and I gave about the science behind biochemical medicine—and possibly twelve attendees—had seen the light.

And one of my autistic patients wanted to grow up to be a nurse in my office!

I headed home after Angie and her mother had left my office, weary with both sorrow and hope. I wanted a glass of cold white wine and a hot bath. I was one raw nerve. I cringed a little when I saw all the cars parked in my driveway when I pulled up to my house. What was going on...?

Oh, right. We were throwing a party.

One of the occupational therapy students who had been studying with Nancy, Dani's therapist, a young Chinese girl named Sabrina, had been delighted to see the piano in our living room the first day she came into our home, and she'd asked if she could play. She was quite accomplished—a talent I appreciated even more because I am musical myself and rarely find the time these days to take much enjoyment from it. I'd asked Sabrina, upon hearing her play that first day, if she'd like us to have a little party where she could play for the guests, and she'd leaped at the idea. I'd forgotten tonight was the night.

My wonderful husband and my magnificent mother once again were executing the plans I had made but hadn't had time to actually do anything about. They had made hors d'oeuvres and were pouring wine for our guests when I walked in. My office family had beat me to my house—though how in the world I had gotten through that day without hearing one of them remind me about this evening... Some of my football players were there with their wives, or girlfriends, or children. My children were there, of course. My son, while passing around a tray of hummus, insisting to anyone who would listen that it be tasted, was showing off pictures of the fuzzy white golden retriever puppy who would grow up to be Dani's service dog, and Dani was perched on the piano bench beside Sabrina while she played. The music was beautiful. Peaceful. My daughter's smile of total engagement and delight in Sabrina's playing was magnificent. My husband handed me a glass of wine and I sank into the rocking chair.

The last few weeks had been dreadful. Wonderful. They had in every way been a strain, and I couldn't think of a better way for them to end, or better people to be around. I felt so tired, but was, for the moment, transported to a place as safe as I wanted to create for Dani—for all my patients. I felt eased. Among my friends, surrounded by the beautiful music, I felt the struggle to get to this safe place end. Just for the evening, but decisively. The safe place, for the next few hours at least, was right here.

Someone started calling for a sing-along. Sabrina asked if there was any sheet music in the house. My son called out, "In the bench," and Sabrina and Dani got up to free the dozens of songbooks in there.

My husband refilled my wine glass as the girls shuffled through the sheet music. The first song they settled down to play—I am not making this up—was "Somewhere over the Rainbow." And we all sang along.

RESOURCES

Where can the parent of an autistic child turn for help? From finding a competent, bio-medically trained physician, to learning the ins and outs of the GFCF diet, to locating parent support groups she can lean on while running the long marathon back to health, our autism community offers a variety of incredible people to consult. Here are some of the places you will find them.

AUTISM SUPPORT RESOURCES

HEAL! (Healing Every Autistic Life)
www.healautismnow.org

HEAL!'s mission is to develop a community and build a HEAL House dedicated to medical research, treatment and education of individuals, community awareness, and, ultimately, prevention of ASDs. I am partial to this organization as I am its co-founder. Among our goals are to provide parent mentors to assist new families who are affected by autism, to train and mentor health care professionals, and to provide parent education seminars as well as social events. We also provide grants to community projects focused on a variety of goals: horse therapy, music education, and special day camps for autistic children.

TACA (Talk About Curing Autism)
www.talkaboutcuringautism.com

At the TACA website you will find listings for local and regional chapters and community events, as well as the opportunity to chat one-on-one online with a TACA parent. Contact with another parent who has experienced a diagnosis of autism is often one of the best ways to glean good advice about how to get your own child started on the journey back to health—and it is darn near always one of the most effective ways of coping for a parent who may, from time to time, find herself overwhelmed on the long road to recovery. The more we connect as a community, sharing knowledge as well as sorrows and joys, the more manageable is our disease on a day-to-day basis.

Also at the TACA website is one of the most concise, practical, and budget-conscious discussions about how to get started on the GFCF diet and the journey into recovery. They have done a beautiful job with this important information, and I highly recommend The Autism Journey Guide as foundational reading.

Healing Our Autistic Children
www.healingourautisticchildren.com
Recognizing that the treatment of autism spectrum disorders is a dynamic, evolving process, this site will be updated frequently, provide links to other resources and ideas as we find them.

FINDING YOUR AUTISM DOCTOR

The National Autism Association
www.nationalautismassociation.org

The Autism Research Institute
www.autism.com

These sites are your resources for finding a local, biomedically trained doctor to treat your child. The Autism Research Institute provides what is currently the most comprehensive list of physicians who have recently received biomedical training. Not everyone who specializes in this approach is listed though, so older practitioners may not be on that list.

Let me say a word or two here about how to go about choosing your biomedical practitioner. Like any physician who guides any patient through any disease, all doctors have varying degrees of expertise in the training they have received. Further, like every other relationship we choose to forge in our lives, the relationship you have with your doctor should be one of mutual respect that allows for the highest degree of clear and honest communication. Do not be afraid to interview doctors to find the one who is right for you and your family. You may find that the first doctor you interview fits this bill—or you may have to interview several to find the one who is the best fit for you and your child. As I have stressed time and again in this book, the journey back to health from a diagnosis of autism is often a lengthy one, and you and the doctor you choose will be together for a long time; take the time to make sure you are comfortable with the doctor's level of expertise, opinions about treatment, and—importantly—"bedside manner."

THE GLUTEN-FREE AND CASEIN-FREE DIET

www.gfcfdiet.com and
www.gfcf.com
These websites are indispensable for those of us on the biomedical path to healing autism. Here you will find the most comprehensive and accurate sources of information about this diet to be found. These sites will likely become ongoing references for every parent—bookmark them.

As I've already noted, TACA's website includes a great deal of good, basic GFCF information too, and the site Healing Our Autistic Children is a resource you can use to vet new discoveries as the science for treating autism spectrum diseases evolves and new discoveries emerge.

GFCF Diet Shopping Cards

The cards below and on the next page are copies of the shopping cards we give to the parents of new patients in my office. Most of the parents find them useful. You can clip these out, laminate them, or fold them in your wallet, and take them to the grocery for easy reference.

These are NOT DAIRY! **They are OKAY!!**	Glycolide
Sodium Lactate	Polylactides
Potassium Lactate	Polyglycolide
Ammonium Lactate	Lactide/glycolide copolymers
Calcium lactate	Gluconates
Aluminum Lactate	Glucono-Delta-Lactone
Ferrous Lactate	Calcium Disodium
Magnesium Lactate	
Zinc Lactate	**Other names for Soy & MSG**
Methyl Lactate	Monoglycerides
Ethyl Lactate	Vegetable Oil/Gum
Isopropyl Lactate	Vitamin E (unless specified as soy-free)
n-Propyl Lactate	Aloe Vera
Butyl Lactate	Lecithin
2-Ethyl-Hexyl Lactate	Natural Flavors
Lactides	MSG (Monosodium Glutamate)
	Soy Oil

SAFE Foods for the GFCF Diet	Quinoa (noodles, flakes & flour)
Fresh fruit	Amaranth
Fresh vegetables	Potato (fresh, starch & flour)
Dried fruit (without sulfites)	Buckwheat flour and groats (Kasha)
Coconut (without sulfites)	Soy (unless intolerant)
Potato chips (plain)	Corn flakes (if specified GF)
Potato sticks	Yams, sweet potatoes (& flours)
Popcorn (NO BUTTER)	Sorghum flour (Jowar)
Rice cakes (check ingredients)	Corn meal (& Polenta)
Rice crackers	Most nuts (unless allergic)
Fresh meat, poultry, fish, shellfish, game	Eggs (unless allergic)
Corn	Beans (& bean flour)
Millet (pilaf and flour)	Lentils
Teff (flour)	Tapioca (Starch)
Rice & rice products (pasta, bread, etc.)	Montina (flour)

Foods to Avoid	Avoid These Additives
Wheat	All aluminum compounds
Bulgar	Artificial colors
Durum	Aspartame (Nutrasweet)
Spelt	BHA, BHT
Triticale	Caffeine
Oats, oat flour	Calcium Disodium EDTA
Barley, barley flour	FD & C colors
Rye	MSG (Monosodium Glutamate)
Semolina (think pasta)	Nitrates, Nitrites
Couscous	Phosphoric Acid
Wheat pasta	Potassium Bromate
Baking powder (unless specified GF)	Quinine
Bouillon cubes or powder	Olestra
Starch, vegetable starch	Polysorbate 60, 80
Sauce mixes (often contain wheat)	Saccharin
Malt, barley malt	Sulfites
Modified food starch	Vanillin (common flavoring)
Rice syrup (unless specified GF, contains barley enzymes)	TBHQ
Spices & herbs (wheat often a filler)	Dextrin (may be derived from wheat)
Artificial colors	

Ingredients that mean DAIRY	
Casein & Caseinates	Cream
Ammonium Caseinate	Curds
Calcium Caseinate	Custard
Magnesium Caseinate	Half & Half
Potassium Caseinate	Sour cream
Sodium Caseinate	Whipped cream
Rennet Casein	
	Milk—in any form
	Non-dairy creamer
Butter	
Artificial butter flavor	Hydrolysates
Butter fat	Casein hydrolysate
Butter flavored oil	Milk protein hydrolysate
Buttermilk	Whey protein hydrolysate
Butter solids	
Whipped butter	Whey—this word in any form!
Cheese	Lactate
Cheese food	Lactic Acid
Cheese flavor	Lactose
ALL types of cheese (hard & soft)	Lactalbumin
Goat cheese	Lactalbumin Phosphate
*Even "non-dairy" cheeses usually have casein!	Sodium Lactylate Lactulose
	Sodium Caseinate
	Sodium Lactylate

REFERENCES

REFERENCES AND ABSTRACTS

These references and abstracts are for the benefit of parents, of course, but my real goal in presenting this section is to provide doctors and other health care providers with a few excerpts of the published scientific literature on which biochemical intervention is predicated. Abstracts are quoted verbatim from source journals. The italicized summaries are my own.

1. Golnik, A., Ireland, M., Borowsky, I.W. 2009. Medical homes for children with autism: a physician survey. *Pediatrics.* 123(3): 966–71.

   This article documents how overwhelmed physicians and pediatricians feel as they face treating autistic children.

   Background: Primary care physicians can enhance the health and quality of life of children with autism by providing high-quality and comprehensive primary care.

   Objective: To explore physicians' perspectives on primary care for children with autism.

   Methods: National mail and e-mail surveys were sent to a random sample of 2325 general pediatricians and 775 family physicians from April 2007 to October 2007.

   Results: The response rate was 19%. Physicians reported significantly lower overall self-perceived competency, a greater need for primary care improvement, and a greater desire for education for children with autism compared with both children with other neurodevelopmental conditions and those with chronic/complex medical conditions. The following barriers to providing primary care were endorsed as greater for children with autism: lack of care coordination, reimbursement and physician education, family skeptical of traditional medicine and vaccines, and patients using complementary alternative medicine. Adjusting for key demographic variables, predictors of both higher perceived autism competency and encouraging an empirically supported therapy, applied behavior analysis, included having a greater number of autism patient visits, having a friend or relative with autism, and previous training about autism.

   Conclusions: Primary care physicians report a lack of self-perceived competency, a desire for education, and a need for improvement in primary care for children with autism. Physician education is needed to improve primary care for children with autism. Practice parameters and models of care should address physician-reported barriers to care.

The following group of papers is about toxicity, how it decreases glutathione, and how nutritional intervention can improve it.

2. Palmer, R., et al. 2006. Environmental mercury release, special education rates, and autism disorder: an ecological study of Texas. *Health and Place.* 12: 203–9.

Abstract: The association between environmentally released mercury, special education and autism rates in Texas was investigated using data from the Texas Education Department and the United States Environmental Protection Agency. A Poisson regression analysis adjusted for school district population size, economic and demographic factors was used. There was a significant increase in the rates of special education students and autism rates associated with increases in environmentally released mercury. On average, for each 1000 lb of environmentally released mercury, there was a 43% increase in the rate of special education services and a 61% increase in the rate of autism. The association between environmentally released mercury and special education rates was fully mediated by increased autism rates. This ecological study suggests the need for further research regarding the association between environmentally released mercury and developmental disorders such as autism. These results have implications for policy planning and cost analysis.

3. James, S.J., et al. 2004. Metabolic biomarkers of increased oxidative stress and impaired methylation capacity in children with autism. *Amer. J. Clin. Nutr.* 80: 1611–17.

The importance of this study is that it demonstrates that children with autism have increased oxidative stress that is measurable and, statistically, significantly worse than in typical children.

Background: Autism is a complex neurodevelopmental disorder that usually develops in early childhood and that is thought to be influenced by genetic and environmental factors. Although abnormal metabolism of methionine and homocysteine has been associated with other neurologic diseases, these pathways have not been evaluated in persons with autism.

Objective: The purpose of this study was to evaluate plasma concentrations of metabolites in the methionine transmethylation and transsulfuration pathways in children diagnosed with autism.

Design: Plasma concentrations of methionine, S-adenosylmethionine (SAM), S-adenosylhomocysteine (SAH), adenosine, homocysteine, cystathionine, cysteine, and oxidized and reduced glutathione were measured in 20 children with autism and in 33 control children. On the basis of the abnormal metabolic profile, a targeted nutritional intervention trial with folinic acid, betaine, and methylcobalamin was initiated in a subset of the autistic children.

Results: Relative to the control children, the children with autism had significantly lower baseline plasma concentrations of methionine, SAM, homocysteine, cystathionine, cysteine, and total glutathione and significantly higher concentrations of SAH, adenosine, and oxidized glutathione. This metabolic profile is consistent with impaired capacity for methylation (significantly lower ratio of SAM to SAH) and increased oxidative stress (significantly lower redox ratio of reduced glutathione to oxidized glutathione) in children with autism. The intervention trial was effective in normalizing the metabolic imbalance in the autistic children.

Conclusion: An increased vulnerability to oxidative stress and a decreased capacity for methylation may contribute to the development and clinical manifestation of autism.

4. Mueller, S.G., et al. 2001. Brain glutathione levels in patients with epilepsy measured by in vivo ^{1}H-MRS. *Neurology*. 57(8): 1422–27.

This study is one example of another disease process that manifests with inadequate glutathione and increased oxidative stress.

Objective: Glutathione in its reduced form (GSH) is the most important free radical scavenging compound in the mammalian nervous system that prevents membrane lipid peroxidation. It is suspected that epileptic seizures are accompanied by a massive production of reactive oxygen species, i.e., oxidative stress.

Results: The GSH/water ratio in patients with epilepsy was significantly reduced in the parietooccipital region of both hemispheres (1.6 +/- 1.0 x 10(−5)) compared to the GSH/water ratio in healthy controls (2.4 +/- 1.1 x 10(−5)). There was no significant difference between the hemisphere with epileptogenic focus and the hemisphere without epileptogenic focus. The GSH/water ratios of the patients without active epilepsy were not different from the GSH/water ratios of patients with active epilepsy.

Conclusion: The authors found evidence for a widespread impairment of the glutathione system in patients with epilepsy independent from seizure activity.

5. James, S.J., et al. March 23, 2009. Cellular and mitochondrial glutathione redox imbalance in lymphoblastoid cells derived from children with autism. *FASEB J.* Epub doi: 10.1096/fj.08–128926.

Dr. James used a cell line from children with autism and exposed the cells to thimerosal (50% mercury by weight). This oxidative stresser resulted in a statistically significant decrease of the autistic cells' ability to produce glutathione when compared with the control group cells.

Abstract: Research into the metabolic phenotype of autism has been relatively unexplored despite the fact that metabolic abnormalities have been implicated in the pathophysiology of several other neurobehavioral disorders. Plasma biomarkers of oxidative stress have been reported in autistic children; however, intracellular redox status has not yet been evaluated. Lymphoblastoid cells (LCLs) derived from autistic children and unaffected controls were used to assess relative concentrations of reduced glutathione (GSH) and oxidized disulfide glutathione (GSSG) in cell extracts and isolated mitochondria as a measure of intracellular redox capacity. The results indicated that the GSH/GSSG redox ratio was decreased and percentage oxidized glutathione increased in both cytosol and mitochondria in the autism LCLs. Exposure to oxidative stress *via* the sulfhydryl reagent thimerosal resulted in a greater decrease in the GSH/GSSG ratio and increase in free radical generation in autism compared to control cells. Acute exposure to physiological levels of nitric oxide decreased mitochondrial membrane potential to a greater extent in the autism LCLs, although GSH/GSSG and ATP concentrations were similarly decreased in both cell lines. These results suggest that the autism LCLs exhibit a reduced glutathione reserve capacity in both cytosol and mitochondria that may compromise antioxidant defense and detoxification capacity under prooxidant conditions.

6. James, S.J., et al. 2009. Efficacy of methylcobalamin and folinic acid treatment on glutathione redox status in children with autism. *Am J Clin Nutr.* 89: 1–6.

    This study shows that the use of methylcobalamin injections and oral folinic acid statistically significantly improved glutathione redox status in children with autism. Mentioned in the paper is that this improvement in redox status correlated with improvement in behavior.

    Background: Metabolic abnormalities and targeted treatment trials have been reported for several neurobehavioral disorders but are relatively understudied in autism.

    Objective: The objective of this study was to determine whether or not treatment with the metabolic precursors, methylcobalamin and folinic acid, would improve plasma concentrations of transmethylation/transsulfuration metabolites and glutathione redox status in autistic children.

    Design: In an open-label trial, 40 autistic children were treated with 75 lg/kg methylcobalamin (2 times/wk) and 400 lg folinic acid (2 times/d) for 3 mo. Metabolites in the transmethylation/transulfuration pathway were measured before and after treatment and compared with values measured in age-matched control children.

    Results: The results indicated that pretreatment metabolite concentrations in autistic children were significantly different from values in the control children. The 3-mo. intervention resulted in significant increases in cysteine, cysteinylglycine, and glutathione concentrations (P, 0.001). The oxidized disulfide form of glutathione was decreased and the glutathione redox ratio increased after treatment (P, 0.008). Although mean metabolite concentrations were improved significantly after intervention, they remained below those in unaffected control children.

    Conclusion: The significant improvements observed in transmethylation metabolites and glutathione redox status after treatment suggest that targeted nutritional intervention with methylcobalamin and folinic acid may be of clinical benefit in some children who have autism.

    This trial was registered at clinicaltrials.gov as NCT00692315.

7. Ziegler, D.R., et al. 2003. Ketogenic diet increases glutathione peroxidase activity in rat hippocampus. *Neurochem Res.* 28(12):1793–97.

    This paper suggests that you can modify oxidative stress and increase glutathione peroxidase through diet.

    Abstract: Ketogenic diets have been used in the treatment of refractory childhood epilepsy for almost 80 years; however, we know little about the underlying biochemical basis of their action. In the hippocampus, however, we observed an increase in antioxidant activity accompanied by an *increase of glutathione peroxidase* (about 4 times) and no changes in lipoperoxidation levels. We suggest that the higher activity of this enzyme induced by ketogenic diet in hippocampus might contribute to protect this structure from neurodegenerative sequelae of convulsive disorders.

The following group of papers weaves together toxic exposures and their impact on the immune system, as well as chronic inflammatory response.

8. Bagenstose, L.M., et al. . 2001. Mercury enhances susceptibility to murine leishmaniasis. *Parasite Immunol.* 23:633–40.

This paper shows that you can take a genetically altered mouse who is normally able to mount an appropriate immune response to (parasitic) infection, expose the mouse to mercury, and suddenly the immunocompetence is lost, and autoimmunity and the allergic processes begin.

Abstract: The genetic background of mice infected with *Leishmania major* determines the response to infection, resulting in a resistant or susceptible phenotype. Susceptible mice develop a T-helper type 2 (Th2)-type immune response following infection distinguished by the development of interleukin (IL)–4 secreting T cells in the lymph node and spleen. In SJL mice, which normally heal *L. major* lesions, subtoxic doses of mercury induce an autoimmune syndrome characterized by an expansion of Th2 cells. In this study, we examined the effect of mercury administration on the outcome of *L. major* infection in SJL mice. We show that subtoxic doses of mercuric chloride ($HgCl_2$) exacerbate disease outcome in SJL mice resulting in increased footpad swelling and increased parasite burdens. Furthermore, the effects of $HgCl_2$ treatment on resistance to *L. major* are time-dependent. The nonhealing phenotype was observed only if mice had been treated with $HgCl_2$ prior to *L. major* infection for at least 1 week, a timepoint at which mice treated with $HgCl_2$ alone had increased splenocyte IL–4 production. $HgCl_2$ treatment also increased production of serum immunoglobulin (Ig)E and IgG1, two IL–4 dependent isotypes. These results show that $HgCl_2$ treatment enhances the susceptibility to *L. major* in SJL mice, consistent with the induction of host Th2 parameters. These findings have implications for the role of mercury contamination in areas of endemic leishmaniasis.

9. Malloy, A.M., et al. 2006. Elevated cytokine levels in children with autism spectrum disorder. *J Neuroimmunol.* 172:198–205.

This paper discusses in complex immunologic terminology that children with autism show immune disregulation.

Abstract: This study compared production of IL–2, IFN-gamma, IL–4, IL–13, IL–5 and IL–10 in peripheral blood mononuclear cells from 20 children with autism spectrum disorder to those from matched controls. Levels of all Th2 cytokines were significantly higher in cases after incubation in media alone, but the IFN-gamma/IL–13 ratio was not significantly different between cases and controls. Cases had significantly higher IL–13/IL–10 and IFN-gamma/IL–10 than controls.

Conclusion: Children with ASD had increased activation of both Th2 and Th1 arms of the adaptive immune response, with a Th2 predominance, and without the compensatory increase in the regulatory cytokine IL–10.

10. Agrawal, A., Kaushal, P., Agrawal, S., Gollapudi, S., Gupta, S. 2007. Thimerosal induces TH2 responses via influencing cytokine secretion by human dendritic cells. *J of Leukoc Biol.* 81: 474–82.

This paper starts by saying that immune dysregulation is induced by mercury and thimerosal and looked for the mechanism by which that happens. The authors found that the immune dysregulation is induced is by the thimerosal, the mercury decreasing glutathione in dendritic (immune) cells.

Abstract: Thimerosal is an organic mercury compound that is used as a preservative in vaccines and pharmaceutical products. Recent studies have shown a TH2-skewing effect of mercury, although the underlying mechanisms have not been identified. In this study, we investigated whether thimerosal can exercise a TH2-promoting effect through modulation of functions of dendritic cells (DC). Thimerosal, in a concentration-dependent manner, inhibited the secretion of LPS-induced proinflammatory cytokines TNF-alpha, IL–6, and IL–12p70 from human monocyte-derived DC. However, the secretion of IL–10 from DC was not affected. These thimerosal-exposed DC induced increased TH2 (IL–5 and IL–13) and decreased TH1 (IFN-gamma) cytokine secretion from the T cells in the absence of additional thimerosal added to the coculture. Thimerosal exposure of DC led to the depletion of intracellular glutathione (GSH), and addition of exogenous GSH to DC abolished the TH2-promoting effect of thimerosal-treated DC, restoring secretion of TNF-alpha, IL–6, and IL–12p70 by DC and IFN-gamma secretion by T cells. These data suggest that modulation of TH2 responses by mercury and thimerosal, in particular, is through depletion of GSH in DC.

11. Vojdani, A. et al. 2008. Low natural killer cell cytotoxic activity in autism: the role of glutathione, IL–2 and IL–15. *J. Neuroimmunol.* doi: 10.1016/ j.jneuroim.2008.09 .005.

This paper discusses more evidence of immune disregulation, in particular with low natural killer (NK) cell activity.

Abstract: Although many articles have reported immune abnormalities in autism, NK cell activity has only been examined in one study of 31 patients, of whom 12 were found to have reduced NK activity. The mechanism behind this low NK cell activity was not explored. For this reason, we explored the measurement of NK cell activity in 1027 blood samples from autistic children obtained from ten clinics and compared the results to 113 healthy controls. This counting of NK cells and the measurement of their lytic activity enabled us to express the NK cell activity/100 cells. At the cutoff of 15–50 LU we found that NK cell activity was low in 41–81% of the patients from the different clinics. This NK cell activity below 15 LU was found in only 8% of healthy subjects (p < 0.001). Low NK cell activity in both groups did not correlate with percentage and absolute number of CD16+/CD56+ cells. When the NK cytotoxic activity was expressed based on activity/100 CD16+/CD56+ cells, several patients who had displayed NK cell activity below 15 LU exhibited normal NK cell activity. Overall, after this correction factor, 45% of the children with autism still exhibited low NK cell activity, correlating with the intracellular level of glutathione. Finally, we cultured lymphocytes of patients with low or high NK cell activity/cell with or without glutathione, IL–2 and IL–15. The induction of NK cell activity by IL–2, IL–15 and glutathione was more pronounced in a subgroup with very low NK cell activity. We conclude that that 45% of a subgroup of children with autism suffers from low NK cell activity, and that low intracellular levels of glutathione, IL–2 and IL–15 may be responsible.

12. Imani, F., Kehoe, K. 2001. Infection of human B lymphocytes with MMR vaccine induces IgE class switching. *Clin Immunol.* 100(3): 355–61.

   This paper shows that a common childhood vaccine may increase potential for allergy.

   Abstract: Circulating immunoglobulin E (IgE) is one of the characteristics of human allergic diseases including allergic asthma. We recently showed that infection of human B cells with rhinovirus or measles virus could lead to the initial steps of IgE class switching. Since many viral vaccines are live viruses, we speculated that live virus vaccines may also induce IgE class switching in human B cells. To examine this possibility, we selected the commonly used live attenuated measles mumps rubella (MMR) vaccine. Here, we show that infection of a human IgM⁺ B cell line with MMR resulted in the expression of germline ε transcript. In addition, infection of freshly prepared human PBLs with this vaccine resulted in the expression of mature IgE mRNA transcript. Our data suggest that a potential side effect of vaccination with live attenuated viruses may be an increase in the expression of IgE.

13. Ashwood, P., et al. 2004. Spontaneous mucosal lymphocyte cytokine profiles in children with autism and gastrointestinal symptoms: mucosal immune activation and reduced counter regulatory interleukin–10. *J Clin Immunol.* 24(6):664–73.

   This paper shows that the disregulation of the immune system extends to intestinal mucosal immunity.

   Abstract: A lymphocytic enterocolitis has been reported in a cohort of children with autistic spectrum disorder (ASD) and gastrointestinal (GI) symptoms. This study tested the hypothesis that dysregulated intestinal mucosal immunity with enhanced pro-inflammatory cytokine production is present in these ASD children. Comparison was made with developmentally normal children with, and without, mucosal inflammation. Duodenal and colonic biopsies were obtained from 21 ASD children, and 65 developmentally normal paediatric controls, of which 38 had signs of histological inflammation. Detection of CD3+ lymphocyte staining for spontaneous intracellular TNFalpha, IL–2, IL–4, IFNgamma, and IL–10, was performed by multicolor flow cytometry. Duodenal and colonic mucosal CD3+ lymphocyte counts were elevated in ASD children compared with noninflamed controls (p<0.03). In the duodenum, the proportion of lamina propria (LP) and epithelial CD3(+)TNFalpha+ cells in ASD children was significantly greater compared with noninflamed controls (p<0.002) but not coeliac disease controls. In addition, LP and epithelial CD3(+)IL–2+ and CD3(+)IFNgamma+, and epithelial CD3(+)IL–4+ cells were more numerous in ASD children than in noninflamed controls (p<0.04). In contrast, CD3(+)IL–10+ cells were fewer in ASD children than in noninflamed controls (p<0.05). In the colon, LP CD3(+)TNFalpha+ and CD3(+)IFNgamma+ were more frequent in ASD children than in noninflamed controls (p<0.01). In contrast with Crohn's disease and non-Crohn's colitis, LP and epithelial CD3(+)IL–10+ cells were fewer in ASD children than in nondisease controls (p<0.01). There was a significantly greater proportion of CD3(+)TNFalpha+ cells in colonic mucosa in those ASD children who had no dietary exclusion compared with those on a gluten and/or casein free diet (p<0.05). There is a consistent profile of CD3+ lymphocyte cytokines in the small and large intestinal mucosa of these ASD children, involving increased pro-inflammatory and decreased regulatory activities. The data provide further evidence of a diffuse mucosal immunopathology in some ASD children and the potential for benefit of dietary and immunomodulatory therapies.

14. Vargas, D., et al. 2004. Neuroglial activation and neuroinflammation in the brain of patients with autism. *Ann of Neurol.* 57 (1): 67–81.

This paper shows evidence of chronic inflammatory processes activated in the brain of patients with autism. The testing was done on brain tissue from the autism brain bank.

Abstract: Autism is a neurodevelopmental disorder characterized by impaired communication and social interaction and may be accompanied by mental retardation and epilepsy. Its cause remains unknown, despite evidence that genetic, environmental, and immunological factors may play a role in its pathogenesis. To investigate whether immune-mediated mechanisms are involved in the pathogenesis of autism, we used immunocytochemistry, cytokine protein arrays, and enzyme-linked immunosorbent assays to study brain tissues and cerebrospinal fluid (CSF) from autistic patients and determined the magnitude of neuroglial and inflammatory reactions and their cytokine expression profiles. Brain tissues from cerebellum, midfrontal, and cingulate gyrus obtained at autopsy from 11 patients with autism were used for morphological studies. Fresh-frozen tissues available from seven patients and CSF from six living autistic patients were used for cytokine protein profiling. We demonstrate an active neuroinflammatory process in the cerebral cortex, white matter, and notably in cerebellum of autistic patients. Immunocytochemical studies showed marked activation of microglia and astroglia, and cytokine profiling indicated that macrophage chemoattractant protein (MCP)–1 and tumor growth factor-1, derived from neuroglia, were the most prevalent cytokines in brain tissues. CSF showed a unique proinflammatory profile of cytokines, including a marked increase in MCP–1. Our findings indicate that innate neuroimmune reactions play a pathogenic role in an undefined proportion of autistic patients, suggesting that future therapies might involve modifying neuroglial responses in the brain.

15. Takashi Ohnishi, et al. 2000. Abnormal regional cerebral blood flow in childhood autism. *Brain.* 123(9): 1838–44.

This paper shows a connection between brain perfusion patterns and brain function abnormalities in autistic patients.

Abstract: Neuroimaging studies of autism have shown abnormalities in the limbic system and cerebellar circuits and additional sites. These findings are not, however, specific or consistent enough to build up a coherent theory of the origin and nature of the brain abnormality in autistic patients. Twenty-three children with infantile autism and 26 non-autistic controls matched for IQ and age were examined using brain-perfusion single photon emission computed tomography with technetium–99m ethyl cysteinate dimer. In autistic subjects, we assessed the relationship between regional cerebral blood flow (rCBF) and symptom profiles. Images were anatomically normalized, and voxel-by-voxel analyses were performed. Decreases in rCBF in autistic patients compared with the control group were identified in the bilateral insula, superior temporal gyri and left prefrontal cortices. Analysis of the correlations between syndrome scores and rCBF revealed that each syndrome was associated with a specific pattern of perfusion in the limbic system and the medial prefrontal cortex. The results confirmed the associations of (i) impairments in communication and social interaction that are thought to be related to deficits in the theory of mind (ToM) with altered perfusion in the medial prefrontal cortex and anterior cingulate gyrus, and (ii) the obsessive desire for sameness with altered perfusion in the right medial temporal lobe. The perfusion abnormalities seem to be related to the cognitive dysfunction observed *in autism,* such as deficits *in* ToM, *abnormal* responses to sensory stimuli, and the obsessive desire for sameness. The perfusion patterns suggest possible locations of abnormalities of brain function underlying abnormal behavior patterns in autistic individuals

16. Benson R.M., et al. 2003. Hyperbaric oxygen inhibits stimulus-induced proinflammatory cytokine synthesis by human blood-derived monocyte-macrophages. *Clin Exp Immunol.* 134(1): 57–62.

This paper, as well as the one after it, shows evidence of the efficacy of hyperbaric treatment. The Benson paper suggests that HBOT has an anti-inflammatory effect.

Abstract: Hyperbaric oxygen (HBO) is 100% oxygen administered at elevated atmospheric pressure to patients with inflammatory diseases. We developed an *in vitro* model to investigate the effects of HBO on stimulus-induced proinflammatory cytokine transcription and translation. Human blood-derived monocytemacrophages were stimulated before being transferred to an HBO chamber where they were incubated at 97·9% O_2, 2·1% CO_2, 2·4 atmospheres absolute, 37∞C. Controls were maintained in the same warm room at normoxia at sea level, hyperoxia or increased pressure alone. A 90-min HBO exposure inhibited IL–1β synthesized in response to lipopolysaccharide by 23%, lipid A by 45%, phytohaemagglutinin A (PHA) by 68%, and tumour necrosis factor (TNF)-α by 27%. HBO suppressed lipopolysaccharide-, lipid A- and PHA-induced TNF-α by 29%, 31% and 62%, respectively. HBO transiently reduced PHA-induced steady state IL–1β mRNA levels. Hyperoxia alone and pressure alone did not affect cytokine production. The immunosuppressive effect of HBO was no longer evident in monocyte-macrophages exposed to HBO for more than 3 h. Interestingly, cells exposed to HBO for 12 h synthesized more IL–1β than cells cultured under control conditions. In summary, HBO exposure transiently suppresses stimulus-induced proinflammatory cytokine production and steady state RNA levels.

17. Rossignol, D., et al. 2009. Hyperbaric treatment for children with autism: a multicenter, randomized, double-blind, controlled trial. *BMC Pediatr.* 9:21. doi:10.1186/1471–2431–9–21.

This paper shows statistically significant improvement in behaviors in children with autism with use of hyperbaric treatment.

Background: Several uncontrolled studies of hyperbaric treatment in children with autism have reported clinical improvements; however, this treatment has not been evaluated to date with a controlled study. We performed a multicenter, randomized, double-blind, controlled trial to assess the efficacy of hyperbaric treatment in children with autism.

Methods: 62 children with autism recruited from 6 centers, ages 2–7 years (mean 4.92±1.21), were randomly assigned to 40 hourly treatments of either hyperbaric treatment at 1.3 atmosphere (atm) and 24% oxygen ("treatment group," n=33) or slightly pressurized room air at 1.03 atm and 21% oxygen ("control group," n=29). Outcome measures included Clinical Global Impression (CGI) scale, Aberrant Behavior Checklist (ABC), and Autism Treatment Evaluation Checklist (ATEC).

Results: After 40 sessions, mean physician CGI scores significantly improved in the treatment group compared to controls in overall functioning (p=0.0008), receptive language (p<0.0001), social interaction (p=0.0473), and eye contact (p=0.0102); 9/30 children (30%) in the treatment group were rated as "very much improved" or "much improved" compared to 2/26 (8%) of controls (p=0.0471); 24/30 (80%) in the treatment group improved compared to 10/26 (38%) of controls (p=0.0024). Mean parental CGI scores significantly improved in the treatment group compared to controls in overall functioning (p=0.0336), receptive language (p=0.0168), and eye contact (p=0.0322). On the ABC, significant improvements were observed in the treatment group in total score, irritability, stereotypy, hyperactivity, and speech (p<0.03 for each), but not in the control group. In the treatment group compared to the control group, mean changes on the ABC total score and subscales were similar except a greater number of children improved in irritability (p=0.0311). On the ATEC, sensory/cognitive awareness significantly improved (p=0.0367) in the treatment group compared to the control group. Post-hoc analysis indicated that children over age 5 and children with lower initial autism severity had the most robust improvements. Hyperbaric treatment was safe and well-tolerated.

Conclusions: Children with autism who received hyperbaric treatment at 1.3 atm and 24% oxygen for 40 hourly sessions had significant improvements in overall functioning, receptive language, social interaction, eye contact, and sensory/cognitive awareness compared to children who received slightly pressurized room air.

OTHER REFERENCES FOR THE PARADIGM THAT CHILDREN WITH AUTISM ARE TREATABLE

The Wakefield and Ashwood papers catalog the nature of the gut disease in autism. The studies by M. Hadjivassiliou discuss gluten sensitivity as causing neurological disease; also note the studies by A.M. Knivsberg that provide evidence of the usefulness of dietary intervention in autism.

Ashwood, P., A. Anthony, et al. 2003. Intestinal lymphocyte populations in children with regressive autism: evidence for extensive mucosal immunopathology. *J Clin Immunol.* 23(6): 504–17.

———. 2004. Spontaneous mucosal lymphocyte cytokine profiles in children with autism and gastrointestinal symptoms: mucosal immune activation and reduced counter regulatory interleukin–10. *J Clin Immunol.* 24(6): 664–73.

Ashwood, P. and A. J. Wakefield. 2006. Immune activation of peripheral blood and mucosal CD3+ lymphocyte cytokine profiles in children with autism and gastrointestinal symptoms. *J Neuroimmunol.* 173(1–2): 126–34.

Baker, B. A., MD, et al. Measuring exposure to an elemental mercury spill—Dakota County, Minnesota, 2004. *MMWR Morb Mortal Wkly Rep.* 54(6): 146–49.

Baskin, D. S., H. Ngo, et al. 2003. Thimerosal induces DNA breaks, caspase–3 activation, membrane damage, and cell death in cultured human neurons and fibroblasts. *Toxicol Sci.* 74(2): 361–68.

Birke, G., A. G. Johnels, et al. 1972. Studies on humans exposed to methyl mercury through fish consumption. *Arch Environ Health.* 25(2): 77–91.

Blaxill, M. F. 2004. What's going on? The question of time trends in autism. *Public Health Rep.* 119(6): 536–51.

Blaxill, M. F., L. Redwood, et al. 2004. Thimerosal and autism? A plausible hypothesis that should not be dismissed. *Med Hypotheses.* 62(5): 788–94.

Bray, T. M. and C. G. Taylor. 1993. Tissue glutathione, nutrition, and oxidative stress. *Can J Physiol Pharmacol.* 71(9): 746–51.

Charleston, J. S., R. L. Body, et al. 1996. Changes in the number of astrocytes and microglia in the thalamus of the monkey Macaca fascicularis following long-term subclinical methylmercury exposure. *Neurotoxicol.* 17(1): 127–38.

Chmelik, E., N. Awadallah, et al. 2004. Varied presentation of PANDAS: a case series. *Clin Pediatr (Phila).* 43(4): 379–82.

Colman, E. 2003. Mercury in infants given vaccines containing thiomersal. *Lancet.* 361(9358): 698; author reply 699.

Croonenberghs, J., E. Bosmans, et al. 2002. Activation of the inflammatory response system in autism. *Neuropsychobiol.* 45(1): 1–6.

Czerucka, D. and P. Rampal. 2002. Experimental effects of *Saccharomyces boulardii* on diarrheal pathogens. *Microbes Infect.* 4(7): 733–39.

Filipek, P. A., P. J. Accardo, et al. 2000. Practice parameter: screening and diagnosis of autism; report of the Quality Standards Subcommittee of the American Academy of Neurology and the Child Neurology Society. *Neurol.* 55(4): 468–79.

Filipek, P. A., J. Juranek, et al. 2003. Mitochondrial dysfunction in autistic patients with 15q inverted duplication. *Ann Neurol.* 53(6): 801–4.

Folstein, S. and M. Rutter. 1977. Genetic influences and infantile autism. *Nature.* 265(5596): 726–28.

Furlano, R. I., A. Anthony, et al. 2001. Colonic CD8 and gamma delta T-cell infiltration with epithelial damage in children with autism. *J Pediatr.* 138(3): 366–72.

Grandjean, P. and P. J. Jorgensen. 2005. Measuring mercury concentration. *Epidemiol.* 16(1): 133.

Gupta, S., S. Aggarwal, et al. 1996. Dysregulated immune system in children with autism: beneficial effects of intravenous immune globulin on autistic characteristics. *J Autism Dev Disord.* 26(4): 439–52.

———. 1998. Th1- and Th2-like cytokines in CD4+ and CD8+ T cells in autism. *J Neuroimmunol.* 85(1): 106–9.

Hadjivassiliou, M., A. Gibson, et al. 1996. Does cryptic gluten sensitivity play a part in neurological illness? *Lancet.* 347(8998): 369–71.

Hadjivassiliou, M., R. A. Grunewald, et al. 2001. Headache and CNS white matter abnormalities associated with gluten sensitivity. *Neurology.* 56(3): 385–88.

Hadjivassiliou, M., R. A. Grunewald, et al. 2002. Gluten sensitivity as a neurological illness. *J Neurol Neurosurg Psychiatry.* 72(5): 560–63.

Hadjivassiliou, M., R. H. Kandler, et al. 2006. Dietary treatment of gluten neuropathy. *Muscle Nerve.* 34(6): 762–66.

Hadjivassiliou, M., D. S. Sanders, et al. 2005. Multiple sclerosis and occult gluten sensitivity. *Neurol.* 64(5): 933–34; author reply 933–34.

Hamilton, R. G. and N. Franklin Adkinson, Jr. 2004. In vitro assays for the diagnosis of IgE-mediated disorders. *J Allergy Clin Immunol.* 114(2): 213–25; quiz 226.

Harding, K. L., R. D. Judah, et al. 2003. Outcome-based comparison of Ritalin versus food-supplement treated children with AD/HD. *Altern Med Rev.* 8(3): 319–30.

Herbert, M. R. 2005. Large brains in autism: the challenge of pervasive abnormality. *Neuroscientist.* 11(5): 417–40.

Herbert, M. R., J. P. Russo, et al. 2006. Autism and environmental genomics. *Neurotoxicol.* 27(5): 671–84.

Hornig, M., H. Weissenbock, et al. 1999. An infection-based model of neurodevelopmental damage. *Proc Natl Acad Sci U S A.* 96(21): 12102–7.

Horvath, K., J. C. Papadimitriou, et al. 1999. Gastrointestinal abnormalities in children with autistic disorder. *J Pediatr.* 135(5): 559–63.

James, S. J., P. Cutler, et al. 2004. Metabolic biomarkers of increased oxidative stress and impaired methylation capacity in children with autism. *Am J Clin Nutr.* 80(6): 1611–17.

Jyonouchi, H., L. Geng, et al. 2005. Dysregulated innate immune responses in young children with autism spectrum disorders: their relationship to gastrointestinal symptoms and dietary intervention. *Neuropsychobiol.* 51(2): 77–85.

Jyonouchi, H., L. Geng, et al. 2005. Evaluation of an association between gastrointestinal symptoms and cytokine production against common dietary proteins in children with autism spectrum disorders. *J Pediatr.* 146(5): 605–10.

Kaplan, B. J., J. McNicol, et al. 1989. Dietary replacement in preschool-aged hyperactive boys. *Pediatr.* 83(1): 7–17.

Kates, W. R., C. P. Burnette, et al. 2004. Frontal and caudate alterations in velocardiofacial syndrome (deletion at chromosome 22q11.2). *J Child Neurol.* 19(5): 337–42.

Knivsberg, A. M. 1997. Urine patterns, peptide levels and IgA/IgG antibodies to food proteins in children with dyslexia. *Pediatr Rehabil.* 1(1): 25–33.

Knivsberg, A. M., K. L. Reichelt, et al. 1995. Autistic symptoms and diet: a follow-up study. *Scand J Ed Res.* 39: 223–36.

Knivsberg, A. M., K. L. Reichelt, et al. 2001. Reports on dietary intervention in autistic disorders. *Nutr Neurosci.* 4(1): 25–37.

Knivsberg, A. M., K. L. Reichelt, et al. 2002. A randomised, controlled study of dietary intervention in autistic syndromes. *Nutr Neurosci.* 5(4): 251–61.

Knivsberg, A. M., K. Wiig, et al. 1990. Dietary intervention in autistic syndromes. *Brain Dysfunction.* 3(5–6): 315–27.

Koch, T. R., L. X. Yuan, et al. 2000. Induction of enlarged intestinal lymphoid aggregates during acute glutathione depletion in a murine model. *Dig Dis Sci.* 45(11): 2115–21.

Levy, S. E., M. C. Souders, et al. 2007. Relationship of dietary intake to gastrointestinal symptoms in children with autistic spectrum disorders. *Biol Psychiatry.* 61(4): 492–97.

Lucarelli, S., T. Frediani, et al. 1995. Food allergy and infantile autism. *Panminerva Med.* 37(3): 137–41.

Magliani, W., S. Conti, et al. 1997. Yeast killer systems. *Clin Microbiol Rev.* 10(3): 369–400.

March, J. S. 2004. Pediatric autoimmune neuropsychiatric disorders associated with strepto-coccal infection (PANDAS): implications for clinical practice. *Arch Pediatr Adolesc Med.* 158(9): 927–29.

Marques, R. C., J. G. Dorea, et al. 2007. Hair mercury in breast-fed infants exposed to thimerosal-preserved vaccines. *Eur J Pediatr.*

McCann, D., A. Barrett, et al. 2007. Food additives and hyperactive behaviour in 3-year-old and 8/9-year-old children in the community: a randomised, double-blinded, placebo-controlled trial. *Lancet.* 370(9598): 1560–67.

McCracken, J. T., J. McGough, et al. 2002. Risperidone in children with autism and serious behavioral problems. *N Engl J Med.* 347(5): 314–21.

Mercer, M. E. and M. D. Holder. 1997. Food cravings, endogenous opioid peptides, and food intake: a review. *Appetite.* 29(3): 325–52.

Messahel, S., A. E. Pheasant, et al. 1998. Urinary levels of neopterin and biopterin in autism. *Neurosci Lett.* 241(1): 17–20.

Millward, C., M. Ferriter, et al. 2004. Gluten- and casein-free diets for autistic spectrum dis-order. *Cochrane Database Syst Rev.* (2): CD003498.

Miraglia del Giudice, M. and M. G. De Luca. 2004. The role of probiotics in the clinical management of food allergy and atopic dermatitis. *J Clin Gastroenterol.* 38(6 Suppl): S84–85.

Mutter, J., J. Naumann, et al. 2005. Mercury and autism: accelerating evidence? *Neuro En-docrinol Lett.* 26(5): 439–46.

Nataf, R., C. Skorupka, et al. 2006. Porphyrinuria in childhood autistic disorder: implications for environmental toxicity. *Toxicol Appl Pharmacol.* 214(2): 99–108.

O'Reilly, B. A. and R. H. Waring. 1993. Enzyme and sulphur oxidation deficiencies in autis-tic children with known food/chemical intolerances. *J Orthomolecular Med.* 8(4): 198–200.

Qvarnstrom, J., L. Lambertsson, et al. 2003. Determination of methylmercury, ethylmercury, and inorganic mercury in mouse tissues, following administration of thimerosal, by species-specific isotope dilution GC-inductively coupled plasma-MS. *Anal Chem.* 75(16): 4120–24.

Panksepp, J. 1979. A neurochemical theory of autism. *Trends Neurosci.* 2: 174–77.

Panksepp, J. and T. L. Sahley. 1987. Possible brain opioid involvement in disrupted social in-tent and language development of autism. *Neurobiological Issues in Autism:* 357–73.

Pelsser, L. M. and J. K. Buitelaar. 2002. [Favorable effect of a standard elimination diet on the behavior of young children with attention deficit hyperactivity disorder (ADHD): a pilot study]. *Ned Tijdschr Geneeskd.* 146(52): 2543–47.

Pelsser, L. M., K. Frankena, et al. 2008. A randomised controlled trial into the effects of food on ADHD. *Eur Child Adolesc Psychiatry.* 35:431–442.

Ramaekers, V. T., J. M. Sequeira, et al. 2008. A milk-free diet downregulates folate receptor autoimmunity in cerebral folate deficiency syndrome. *Dev Med Child Neurol.* 50(5): 346–52.

Ramirez, G. B., M. C. Cruz, et al. 2000. The Tagum study I: analysis and clinical correlates of mercury in maternal and cord blood, breast milk, meconium, and infants' hair. *Pediatr.* 106(4): 774–81.

Rampersad, G. C., G. Suck, et al. 2005. Chemical compounds that target thiol-disulfide groups on mononuclear phagocytes inhibit immune mediated phagocytosis of red blood cells. *Transfusion.* 45(3): 384–93.

Reichelt, K. L., J. Ekrem, et al. 1990. Gluten, milk proteins and autism: dietary intervention effects on behavior and peptide secretion. *J Appl Nutr.* 42(1): 1–11.

Reichenberg, A., R. Yirmiya, et al. 2001. Cytokine-associated emotional and cognitive disturbances in humans. *Arch Gen Psychiatry.* 58(5): 445–52.

Richardson, A. J. 2006. Omega–3 fatty acids in ADHD and related neurodevelopmental disorders. *Int Rev Psychiatry.* 18(2): 155–72.

Rimland, B. 2000. Secretin treatment for autism. *N Engl J Med.* 342(16): 1216–17; author reply 1218.

Rogers, S. J. 1996. Brief report: early intervention in autism. *J Autism Dev Disord.* 26(2): 243–46.

Rossignol, D. A. and L. W. Rossignol. 2006. Hyperbaric oxygen therapy may improve symptoms in autistic children. *Med Hypotheses.* 67(2): 216–28.

Snider, L. A. and S. E. Swedo. 2004. PANDAS: current status and directions for research. *Mol Psychiatry.* 9(10): 900–7.

Stajich, G. V., G. P. Lopez, et al. 2000. Iatrogenic exposure to mercury after hepatitis B vaccination in preterm infants. *J Pediatr.* 136(5): 679–81.

Stern, A. H. 2005. A revised probabilistic estimate of the maternal methyl mercury intake dose corresponding to a measured cord blood mercury concentration. *Environ Health Perspect.* 113(2): 155–63.

Stevens, L. J., S. S. Zentall, et al. 1995. Essential fatty acid metabolism in boys with attention-deficit hyperactivity disorder. *Am J Clin Nutr.* 62(4): 761–68.

Stoller, K. P. 2005. Quantification of neurocognitive changes before, during, and after hyperbaric oxygen therapy in a case of fetal alcohol syndrome. *Pediatr.* 116(4): e586–91.

Sturniolo, G. C., V. Di Leo, et al. 2001. Zinc supplementation tightens leaky gut in Crohn's disease. *Inflamm Bowel Dis.* 7(2): 94–98.

Swedo, S. E., H. L. Leonard, et al. 1998. Pediatric autoimmune neuropsychiatric disorders associated with streptococcal infections: clinical description of the first 50 cases. *Am J Psychiatry.* 155(2): 264–71.

Swedo, S. E., H. L. Leonard, et al. 1997. Identification of children with pediatric autoimmune neuropsychiatric disorders associated with streptococcal infections by a marker associated with rheumatic fever. *Am J Psychiatry.* 154(1): 110–12.

Torrente, F., A. Anthony, et al. 2004. Focal-enhanced gastritis in regressive autism with features distinct from Crohn's and *Helicobacter pylori* gastritis. *Am J Gastroenterol.* 99(4): 598–605.

Torrente, F., P. Ashwood, et al. 2002. Small intestinal enteropathy with epithelial IgG and complement deposition in children with regressive autism. *Mol Psychiatry.* 7(4): 375–82, 334.

Valicenti-McDermott, M., K. McVicar, et al. 2006. Frequency of gastrointestinal symptoms in children with autistic spectrum disorders and association with family history of autoimmune disease. *J Dev Behav Pediatr.* 27(2 Suppl): S128–36.

Vancassel, S., G. Durand, et al. 2001. Plasma fatty acid levels in autistic children. *Prostaglandins Leukot Essent Fatty Acids.* 65(1): 1–7.

Vargas, D. L., C. Nascimbene, et al. 2005. Neuroglial activation and neuroinflammation in the brain of patients with autism. *Ann Neurol.* 57(1): 67–81.

Vojdani, A., T. O'Bryan, et al. 2004. Immune response to dietary proteins, gliadin and cerebellar peptides in children with autism. *Nutr Neurosci.* 7(3): 151–61.

Wakefield, A. J., A. Anthony, et al. 2000. Enterocolitis in children with developmental disorders. *Am J Gastroenterol.* 95(9): 2285–95.

Wakefield, A. J., S. H. Murch, et al. 1998. Ileal-lymphoid-nodular hyperplasia, non-specific colitis, and pervasive developmental disorder in children. *Lancet.* 351(9103): 637–41.

Warren, R. P., A. Foster, et al. 1987. Reduced natural killer cell activity in autism. *J Am Acad Child Adolesc Psychiatry.* 26(3): 333–35.

Warren, R. P., N. C. Margaretten, et al. 1986. Immune abnormalities in patients with autism. *J Autism Dev Disord.* 16(2): 189–97.

Werner, E. and G. Dawson. 2005. Validation of the phenomenon of autistic regression using home videotapes. *Arch Gen Psychiatry.* 62(8): 889–95.

Woods, J. S. 1996. Altered porphyrin metabolism as a biomarker of mercury exposure and toxicity. *Can J Physiol Pharmacol.* 74(2): 210–15.

Woods, J. S., D. L. Eaton, et al. 1984. Studies on porphyrin metabolism in the kidney. Effects of trace metals and glutathione on renal uroporphyrinogen decarboxylase. *Mol Pharmacol.* 26(2): 336–41.

Woods, J. S., M. D. Martin, et al. 1993. Urinary porphyrin profiles as a biomarker of mercury exposure: studies on dentists with occupational exposure to mercury vapor. *J Toxicol Environ Health.* 40(2–3): 235–46.

Woods, J. S. and H. D. Miller. 1993. Quantitative measurement of porphyrins in biological tissues and evaluation of tissue porphyrins during toxicant exposures. *Fundam Appl Toxicol.* 21(3): 291–97.

Wright, C. E., H. H. Tallan, et al. 1986. Taurine: biological update. *Annu Rev Biochem.* 55: 427–53.

Yokoo, E. M., J. G. Valente, et al. 2003. Low level methylmercury exposure affects neuropsychological function in adults. *Environ Health.* (1): 8.

INDEX